MW00445473

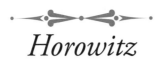

Horowitz

LOVE The Real Da Vinci CODE

Maximizing Your Creative Genius, Health, and Wealth Through Divine Communion

by

Dr. Leonard G. Horowitz

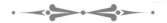

Tetrahedron, LLC

Cover designed by Len Horowitz
Manufactured in the United States of America

10 9 8 7 6 5 4 3 2 1

Library of Congress Cataloging Preassigned
Horowitz, Leonard G.
    LOVE The Real Da Vinci CODE
    p.   cm.
    Includes bibliographical references.
    1. Popular Works;
      —Personal development
      —Self-help
    3. Energy medicine—Mathematics
      —Alternative medicine—Physics
      —Water science—Bioenergetics
    5. Spiritual healing

2. Philosophy/Religion
  —Intelligent design—Creationism

4. New Age/Judeo-Christian theology

Card Number: Pending
Additional cataloging data pending.

ISBN: 0-923550-66-6
ISBN 13: 978-0-923550-66-0

Additional copies of this book are available for bulk purchases.
For more information, please contact:
Tetrahedron, LLC • Suite 147, 206 North 4th Avenue • Sandpoint, Idaho 83864,
1-888-508-4787; E-mail: tetra@tetrahedron.org,

URL web site: http://www.tetrahedron.org

First printing

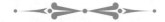

LOVE The Real Da Vinci CODE

Illustrations

Course Objectives

Chapters

About the author

References and Notes

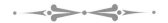

Illustrations

Figures

Tables

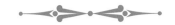

LOVE *The Real Da Vinci* CODE

Objectives of this Book:

By the end of this course, you should develop:

• **Content knowledge**—an understanding of math in creative language, music, art and science and the use of simple musical-mathematics to recreate your life and fulfill your Divine destiny;

• **Structural knowledge**—an understanding of ideas advanced by Leonardo Da Vinci, and his predecessors Plato and Pythagoras, pertaining to creative mathematics, related creationistic science, and the laws governing the physical world from the spiritual domain;

• **Historical context**—interpretations of languages as they relate to history, math, and music;

• **Critical thinking**—appreciation of the advancement of creative "out of the box" reasoning; how human communications operate to compel miraculous manifestations "either good or bad" affecting your life and civilization's communion;

• **Technical reading**—of ancient mystery school mathematics, sacred geometrics, and related life skills;

• **Appreciation for the beauty of nature**—as sacred architecture involving simple mathematics from whence everything comes);

• **Instructional Methods and Activities**—includes daily exercises, personal processes, and fill-in-the-blank instructions; reading assignments; expanding Divine–Self Evaluation, and ongoing self-examination.

Chapter 1.

Introduction to the Real Code

Where is the code in *The Da Vinci Code*? You won't find the biggest secret in the book or movie.

By definition, a code is, "a system of signals . . . or symbols used for brevity or secrecy of communication . . . ; a systematic collection of the existing laws . . . ; [and] any system of principles."

Leonardo da Vinci was inspired by a secret, sacred, powerful code that has remained hidden until now. This book decrypts that code and explains why it has remained hidden.

LOVE The Real Da Vinci Code can help you express your creative genius, improve your health, and even gain wealth. What is this awesome intelligence worth?

This optimally-empowering revelation is great news if you desire to reveal your greatest good and hidden talents, and switch your success-rate into hyper drive. Pay special attention to what you are about to learn.

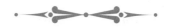

LOVE *The Real Da Vinci* CODE

The code decrypted here is unlike any other. It was created by the universal Master of creation to empower and sustain everyone and everything. It is also used to administer "Divine Justice" granting what you choose consciously and subconsciously. The code is revealed herein to inspire your creative genius and the restoration, evolution, and sustenance of life on this planet.

Chapter 2.
Breaking the Code of Da Vinci

In June 2006, during a trip to South Africa, while confronted with my inability to alter the course of AIDS history, I asked our Creator for reassurance concerning my perceived insignificance. An inner voice replied saying, "You have a very important role to play in the great healing of the nations." Then, a vision of Da Vinci's Vitruvian Man spontaneously captured my imagination. In that instant the Creator showed me the universal technology inspiring creative genius for recreating our planet and solving the AIDS crisis and every other problem confronting the world today.

The technology governing spiritual power to recreate ourselves in the image of God was included in this gift of insight. The Vitruvian Man, I realized, was a cryptograph mapping God's core creative technology. This capability—the code— is characterized by the secret sacred principles, signals, symbols, and laws that compel creative genius.

Leonardo da Vinci was illuminated and inspired by this knowledge. History's greatest Renaissance Man moved mountains in the arts and sciences because

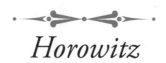

of this intelligence. His prophetic visions generated many of history's most beautiful, brilliant, scientific, technical, and imaginative achievements. His loving labors epitomized The Universal Man, and his revelations had global implications for sustaining, remaking, and advancing civilization.

Due to the implications of these revelations, *LOVE The Real Da Vinci Code* is more than a book. This is a global project. This precious effort makes Da Vinci's special intelligence and inspiration available to everyone. It calls you to do what Leonardo did as a master of metaphysics and commander of spiritual dynamics, that is, use your creative capacity to serve humanity.

This work is, therefore, dedicated to Da Vinci and to the Renaissance Man in you. My overall objective is to advance knowledge that can be used to dramatically improve life on our precious Earth.

I have earned several academic degrees, contributed many scientific publications, written fifteen published books and produced dozens of DVDs and CDs over the past twenty years. (See: www.DrLen-Horowitz.com) *LOVE the Real Da Vinci Code* compiles much of this knowledge and research. Most importantly, in 1998, I wrote *Healing Codes for the*

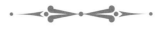

LOVE The Real Da Vinci CODE

Biological Apocalypse prompted by Dr. Joseph Puleo, who instructed me to begin decrypting codes in music, mathematics, and languages.

More important than my academic training, however, is the critical direction I received for this project from the spiritual realm. There are forces in nature, that I gratefully and humbly acknowledge and conclude, represents a Divine hand.

I proclaim a Divine hand in this direction partly to test your discernment. More important than what I believe is what you receive. As you read this book, check if you perceive the fruit of this labor as savory and sweet as it applies to your life.

Nearly five thousand years ago master Masons applied this code to design and build some of the world's most amazing architectural wonders, including the Great Pyramid of Giza. Temples were similarly constructed according to this sacred knowledge of mathematics, music, and spiritually-conductive design. The dimensions of King Solomon's Temple in the Holy Land were calculated according to this code. The Bible records these dimensions evidencing this code's application. Suffice it to say Leonardo da Vinci was not the first to acquire this Divine technology.

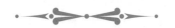

LOVE The Real Da Vinci CODE

By understanding the Da Vinci code, you are presented with a Divine invitation for spiritual evolution, universal unification, and planetary salvation.

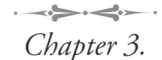

Chapter 3.
Your Required Investment

To assimilate this extraordinary metaphysically-empowering information, and have it work for you, you will need to make a reasonable investment of your own time and money. You will learn why this is necessary—including the mathematical mechanism behind this—in the pages ahead.

Simply recognizing the sanctity of this knowledge compels a responsible investment, and there is no need to fear, your investments in this opportunity will be rewarded.

Likewise, by sharing this most powerful creative technology with you, my investment in you shall be rewarded. The Law you will learn about demands an equitable return on our investments in each other.

In ancient times, priests never asked to be paid for their wisdom or services since they operated according to the Divine Law of tithing. People benefitted from their counsel and simply donated a reasonable portion of their first fruit—the best of their harvest, livestock, or wealth. In return people were spiritually blessed and physically sustained.

This is not always practiced in today's world although the Law continues in the spiritual realm.

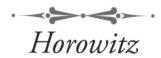

This project engages the Creator's realm of spirit and provides general access to it. Thus, creatively operating here demands continuous "giving back" or "paying it forward." That is, for you to regain and maintain the real Da Vinci code's miraculous enabling power you will need to contribute, perhaps more than you ever have, to our ministry affiliates.

Consensus among Bible scholars holds that nine (9) percent of first fruits will satisfy a tithe. To proceed enabled by the spiritually-empowering, life-changing, metaphysical revelations continued herein you must feel comfortable about *tithing*. You also need to feel favorable about receiving, and following, higher spiritual direction. This investment, and program, forms far more than a partnership with me as your guide. This "magical-mystery tour" will continue to bear fruit multiplied for many others served by our investments because this rule of multiplication is established by Law.

You are about to consider this Law in the pages ahead. Miracles manifest in compliance with this system of justice. Alternatively, the Law will prohibit your further progress, and optimal success, if you fail your test, that is, you fail to invest your heart, time, and nine percent. This is an exacting Law that is certified by science and ancient scripture.

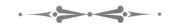

LOVE *The Real Da Vinci* CODE

It's obviously wise to put your heart and time into important projects. But, why is only nine percent of your increased income demanded here?

Here is your answer:

You will undoubtedly increase your creative output and, if you intend, generate more wealth by applying this creative knowledge and technology in your life and career. The Provider of this knowledge has contracted to multiply your return on this investment. This serves everyone, including the Source of this blessing who wishes to sustain you, and other kindred spirits, in joy and prosperity. This is administered using the fundamental mathematics discussed herein; energizing dynamics upon which this successful partnership can continue. This Law is certified by both Old and New Testaments in the Bible as well as modern, and ancient mystery school, teachings.

In other words, there is a historically-proven Levitical covenant and wealth building dynamic that requires the tithe. I am the Levite appointed to remind you of this and advance this math and planet-wide project.

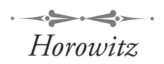

A convenient way to think about this was suggested by John D. Hendricks in his book *Prosperity God's Way*. "People seem to have no problem as to how God set up life to provide for man," Hendricks, a minister, wrote. "You can sow a few thousand seeds and they will grow into millions more, like a cornfield. . . . No one has difficulty believing and conceiving farming. Yet it seems to be difficult for people to believe that when they give of their finances, God will do the same thing, but He does."

Jesus's adversary turned apostle, Paul, wrote in II Corinthians 9:6-8, "But this I say, He that sows sparingly shall reap also sparingly; and he that sows bountifully shall reap also bountifully." Every man according to the purpose in his heart, should give; "not grudgingly, or of necessity: for God loveth a cheerful giver. And God is able to make all grace abound toward you; that ye, always having all sufficiency in all things, may abound to every good work."

LOVE The Real Da Vinci Code is, indeed, one such good work. So rejoice expecting the greatest blessings from it. Minister Hendricks concludes, "When you abundantly share properly, it gives God the freedom, the legal right, to move for you in this world."

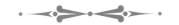

LOVE The Real Da Vinci CODE

You are about to learn how and why this happens—the precise mathematics and scientific understanding underlying this truth. *LOVE The Real Da Vinci Code* reveals how the universe works to affect this and all spiritual dynamics, including all metaphysics. All of this is a result of *giving and receiving*. These two seemingly opposite verbs, this code explains, are really the *same*.

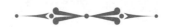

Chapter 4.
The Missing Code in
The Da Vinci Code

Dan Brown developed the popular, highly controversial, novel from which a thrilling film was made. Both book and movie featured glimpses of Leonardo da Vinci's magnificent art and mysterious life. More than 25 million copies of *The Da Vinci Code*, in 44 languages, have been circulated to date; all revealing virtually nothing about the real code that made the Renaissance Man a creative genius.

In fact, the only use of a mathematical code in *The Da Vinci Code* came near the beginning of the book. Princess Sophie rejected Fibonacci's series of numbers—1, 1, 2, 3, 5, 8, 13, 21—as meaningless to her investigation of her grandfather's murder.

In addition, The Vitruvian Man is only fleetingly mentioned in *The Da Vinci Code*. It presented a personal message to the heroin of the book to recruit her engagement in an investigation of secret-societies, one of which was protecting her.

Based on the unifying truths revealed herein, the controversy sparked by *The Da Vinci Code* centering on Jesus's alleged offspring, and the sacred feminine suppression by organized religion, may be seen as symptomatic of a deeper pathology—*ignorance of*

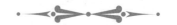

this code. In health science this illness is labeled a "social scatoma." The widespread myopic disorder results in estrangement of humans from our Divine family. This spiritually-incapacitating imposition of organized religion and sovereignty-assailing governments yields superficial chronically-divisive debates, even wars, inconsistent with the unifying technology heralded here.

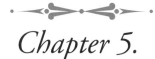

Chapter 5.
Facts About Creative Mathematics

Leonardo da Vinci was incredibly prophetic and precisely visionary primarily as a result of having received a "Master Code" for applied wisdom. This code had been passed down through the ages. Da Vinci's heroes, Plato and Pythagoras, were privy to it. "The Lost Temple Code" or "Genius Code" demystifies the Creator's primary laws of creation. It advances the world's most powerful creationistic technology. *The real Da Vinci code is the Source Code for enlightenment, unleashing human genius, and the creative power to manifest miracles in the real world.*

As a result of obtaining this knowledge, the Renaissance Man habitually encoded his research notes and wrote backwards! Why? Not simply for secrecy, although this has been alleged by many scholars. He wrote "back*words*" because of his knowledge of the creative dynamics of language, its underlying polarity or mirrored mathematics, and the impact of balancing left/right brain function.

To be optimally creative, intuitive, and resourceful, you need to balance, integrate, and develop both hemispheres of your brain. Your left brain is more rational and scientific. Your right brain is consid-

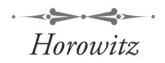
ered more imaginative and intuitive. Developing and integrating both sides of your brain, so that they both work together, is central to learning creative language, processing information, and receiving wisdom for life mastery.

In fact, everything in the universe is based on math. This includes the creative power of language. Language is math because sound is electromagnetic frequencies, and that is math. Language and sounds are heard because they vibrate at certain rates called Hertz frequencies, or cycles per second. Your brain perceives these energized vibrations, this math, much like your ears hear music from vibrations. Your brain interprets these messages according to your programming, that is, your neurology and memory circuits formed from life experiences. Much like 1950s or 60s music triggers memories for those who lived them, the ancient math presented here can trigger knowledge or wisdom from times long gone and also forthcoming. Future vision is due to the proven concept of space/time relativity, which is also based on simple mathematics and laws of physics you are about to consider.

So math, as you will increasingly integrate in this interactive program, is the basis of everything.

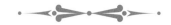

LOVE *The Real Da Vinci* CODE

The Magic of Math in Language

Each letter of the alphabet carries a certain frequency of sound or energy. That is, a certain set of mathematical vibrations—cycles per second—underlies communication in all languages. This is expressed in numbers for each letter. So there is an alpha-numeric, that is, letter/number basis for all languages and verbal communications that your brain interprets for better or worse.

According to acoustics and linguistics scholars, a language's alpha-numerics, and ability to affect human consciousness, are two characteristics of sacred languages such as Hebrew and Sanskrit.

Da Vinci studied the musical-mathematical teachings of architectural masters including Pythagoras, Plato and Vitruvius. He applied the encoded alpha-numeric ancient sacred languages during work and play to expand his capacity to access the mathematical Matrix of space/time. This is detailed in Chapter 14.

From his study and practice, The Renaissance Man was able to access the creative power available in the Matrix—also called the "Kingdom of Heaven" in the religious world. All of this is exquisitely represented in his famous drawings, especially The Vitruvian

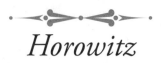
Man which will be discussed at length later.

To support this thesis, I quote from expert Graham Pont's outstanding research report, "Philosophy and Science of Music in Ancient Greece: Predecessors of Pythagoras and their Contribution," published in *Nexus Network Journal* (vol. 6, no. 1; 2004). This peer-reviewed scholarly periodical delves into the mathematics of music, other creative arts, and the sciences:

> "[T]he Pythagorean vision of the living cosmos—or Plato's 'World Soul'—has reappeared in new vitalist theories, . . . The modern world-view and its vast astronomical time-frame have changed our conception of humanity itself, . . . The integers 6, 8, 9 and 12 are the smallest whole numbers with which the symmetrical system of interlocking ratios—the natural framework of the ancient and modern diatonic scales—can be expressed. . . . Plato characterized the good man as 'living 729 times more pleasantly, and the tyrant more painfully by this same interval' (Republic 587e). . . .

Plato's model here is both musical and geometrical; 729 decodes to 9 as you will soon learn.

> "Similarly [Ernest] McClain decoded many other musical allegories and discovered the meaning of some incredibly large numbers in Babylonian, Egyptian, Hindu, Greek, and Hebrew texts. In *The Pythagorean Plato*, he applied the same method to Plato's numerology and produced a simple, consistent and comprehensive expla-

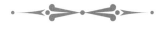
nation of allegorical texts that had defeated five hundred years of classical scholarship. . . .

"The key to Plato's musico-political analogies is here revealed for the first time, . . . with a whole gamut of harmonic terms resonating through the European languages." [Spitzer, 1963]

In other words, math, music, and language go hand in hand with everything from politics to profits.

As strange as this may seem, civilizations are built on the musical-mathematics of language. More strange than this, some Western languages, such as English, have been alpha-numerically *reversed*.

Given this knowledge, to reverse his mixed mathematical messaging affecting brain function, Da Vinci wrote sbɿɒwʞɔɒd, or "backwords."

He made it a game. With this heart for fun and fundamentals—this balanced orientation, expanded mathematical mind, and super-charged neurology—he gained superior intuitive reception, prophetic vision, and many masterful skills.

While the rest of humanity struggled for survival in the Dark Ages, Da Vinci mathematically exercised both hemispheres of his brain to develop his superhuman creative talents.

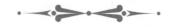

LOVE *The Real Da Vinci* CODE

You can and may do this too, given this simple know-how and routine practice.

Chapter 6.
Important Da Vinci Definitions

To cement this language lesson in your mind consider these definitions. According to historians, Da Vinci was a master of "polymath," "polyhistor," and "mathema."

Polymath sources from the Greek word *polys*, meaning "much," or "great in quantity;" and *mathese* meaning "learning." So a person who excels in multiple fields, particularly both arts and sciences is a master of polymath.

Polyhistor is a synonym for polymath. In fact, histor and math mean the same: "knowledge, learn, or learned." Histor implies erudition and wisdom. Erudition means "the scholarly achievement from instruction and reading followed by assimilation and contemplation that efface all rudeness; smoothes-away all the raw and untrained incivility. It is the depth, polish, and breadth that is applied to education."

The word education, derives from the Latin word *educare* which means to "lead out from within."

The word history, or histor with the "e" symbol for energy, implies knowledge of energy and the math-

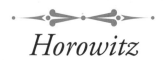

ematics fundamental to energetics. Both of these are timeless, eternal, and fundamental to everything.

Philomath means "a lover of learning." Plato and Aristotle defined mathema as relative to *disciplina* (discipline); *doctrina* (learning the fundamental laws governing everything); and *cognitio* (cognition) or understanding the universe and the fundamental mathematical basis for the cosmos. These philosophers, and their many disciples, considered mathema in terms of education; which included arithmetic, geometry, astronomy, and music.

Leonardo da Vinci is quoted as saying: "There is no certainty where one cannot apply any of the mathematical sciences." Universal certainty, divine/human unity, and co-creativity is established by math. The road to finding oneself, including your highest qualities and greatest creative potentials, is paved by mystery school math.

You are about to learn the secret sacred principles, signals, symbols, and laws that shall set you free.

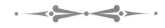
EXERCISES:

1) To introduce yourself to ancient mystery-school mathematics complete the figure on the next page. Reduce each double digit to the Pythagorean single digit integer.

2) Read the following reversed message. If you need help, use a mirror:

The end of shadow-governors control is chosen. Millennia of malicious manipulation nears termination. Servants of injustice shall perish. The Matrix dictates earthly renewal.

3) Consider the Fibonacci Series of numbers: 1 1 2 3 5 8 13 21. Add all these numbers and reduce to a single digit. What number do you get for completion?

$$1 + 1 + 2 + 3 + 5 + 8 + 13 + 21$$
$$2 \quad 5 \quad 13 \quad 34$$
$$7 \quad + \quad 47$$
$$54 = 9$$

1 1 2 3 5 8 13 21

Table 1. Pythagorean Numbering System

EVEN/LEFT COLUMN (Odd or Even Result)	ODD/RIGHT COLUMN (Even or Odd Result)
10 = 1 + 0 = 1	11 = 1 + 1 = 2
12 = 1 + 2 = 3	13 = 1 + 3 = 4
14 = 1 + 4 = 5	15 = 1 + 5 = 6
16 = 1 + 6 = 7	17 = _ + 7 = 8
18 = 1 + 8 = 9	19 = 1 + 9 = 10
20 = 2 + 0 = 2	21 = 2 + 1 = 3
22 = 2 + 2 = 4	23 = 2 + 3 = 5
24 = 2 + 4 = 6	25 = 2 + 5 = 7
26 = 2 + 6 = 8	27 = 2 + 7 = 9
30 = 3 + 0 = 3	31 = 3 + 1 = 4
32 = 3 + 2 = 5	33 = 3 + 3 = 6
34 = 3 + 4 = 7	35 = 3 + 5 = 8
36 = 3 + 6 = 9	

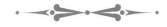

4) **A major event occurs in the Bible in Revelation 14:1. Look this up and answer the following questions:**

a. **The Lamb stands on what? Do you recognize this name from *The Da Vinci Code?*** Mont Zion

b. **What number of people sing for "completion" in the End Times?** 144,000

c. **Where is the "Father's name" written? Why here?** FOREHEAD   classification

d. **In Rev. 14:2 the "voice from heaven" is as the voice of many what?** WATERS

5) **Sound/math energy placed in water is fundamental to creation. Go online to http://www.liveh2o.org to collaborate in recreating our world.**

6) Read the following message and answer the question it poses:

In ancient times buildings were designed and constructed by master Masons schooled in the math you are learning here. They measured all assignments using cut reeds. The standard measuring reed was trimmed to precisely 6 cubits and 1 handbreath called a great cubit. A standard cubit was 6 handbreaths; again, 7 handbreaths for great cubits. So the measuring reed measured 6x7=42 handbreaths. Converted to modern measures a full reed was 12 feet, 6 inches. Typically, Bible constructions, such as the ancient temples and Noah's ark, were designed respecting three special numbers. Using the information above, and Bible verse building descriptions, determine these three numbers now. What are these numbers?

4 6 7   369

Chapter 7
The Alpha-Numeric Code and Language Creation

The book *Healing Codes for the Biological Apocalypse* has been inspiring musicians and mathematicians worldwide. The book was prompted by Bible code revelations—how mathematics, the most precise language, is God's language because it always speaks the truth.

I learned that the Hebrew language, as well as English backwards, held a spiritual relationship with the Creator. In fact, all sacred languages have been mathematically designed to advance creative consciousness and Divine spirituality.

To prove this little-known point, and develop your left-brain/right-brain balance as Da Vinci did, take the English alphabet and number each letter. For example, A=1, B=2, C=3, and so on, as seen in Table 2. Notice, when the two digit numbers are reduced to their single digit numbers, as routinely performed in mystery-school math, this results in a pattern of 1 thru 9, 1 thru 9, and 1 thru 8.

In mystery school, Pythagoras taught there are only 9 numbers in the universe: 1–9; with 9 symbolizing

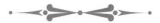

Table 2. Derivation of English Letter Number Code

Letter & Number	Pythagorean Skein Equivalent	Key Word Number Derivations
A 1	1	T 20–2 + 0 = 2
B 2	2	R 18–1 + 8 = 9
C 3	3	U 21–2 + 1 = 3
D 4	4	S 19–1 + 9 = 1
E 5	5	T 20–2 + 0 = 2
F 6	6	98=8 17=8
G 7	7	
H 8	8	
I 9	9	F 6–6 + 0 = 6
J 10	1 + 0 = 1	A 1–1 + 0 = 1
K 11	1 + 1 = 2	I 9–9 + 0 = 9
L 12	1 + 2 = 3	T 20–2 + 0 = 2
M 13	1 + 3 = 4	H 8–8 + 0 = 8
N 14	1 + 4 = 5	44=8 26=8
O 15	1 + 5 = 6	
P 16	1 + 6 = 7	G 7–7 + 0 = 7
Q 17	1 + 7 = 8	O 15–1 + 5 = 6
R 18	1 + 8 = 9	D 4–4 + 0 = 4
S 19	1 + 9 = 10	26=8 17=8
T 20	2 + 0 = 2	
U 21	2 + 1 = 3	The number 8
V 22	2 + 2 = 4	represents
W 23	2 + 3 = 5	Divinity & infinity.
X 24	2 + 4 = 6	9 represents
Y 25	2 + 5 = 7	completion.
Z 26	2 + 6 = 8	

Table shows the English alphabet and its equivalent numbers. Two or more digit numbers are reduced to single digit numbers to employ the Pythagorean skein and determine the mathematical "truth." Notice that numbers one through nine repeat; and the number 8, the universal sign for infinity, is also the total for Trust, Faith and God. The number nine (9) represents completion. Excerpted from *Walk on Water* (Tetrahedron, LLC, 2006).

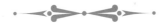
completion. 10 is really 1 + 0, which is 1. The 0 is not a number. Zeros are recognized as being place holders. But more than this, a "place holder" for all numbers is virtually the "Kingdom of Heaven." Zero symbolizes nothing, and simultaneously, the whole ring or circle of everything, like the "Circle of Life." You will learn more about this concept in the coming pages.

When you perform a mathematical translation on the words TRUST, FAITH, and GOD, the same sum total of 8 occurs.

For TRUST, T=20 + R=18 + U=21, + S=19 + T=20 totals 98. Then reduce 98 to a single digit—9+8=17; then finally, 1+7=8.

For FAITH, F=6, A=1, I=9, T=20, and H=8 totals 44. And 4+4=8.

For GOD, G=7, O=15, and D=4 totals 26. And again 2+6=8.

Eight (8) is the sign of infinity, that is, God's number. It is also the number for oxygen in the periodic table of elements. Interesting because the Hebrew name for God—Yod-Hey-Vov-Hey, or Yah for short—means "to breathe is to exist." Fascinating also because to animate Adam, humanity's first born,

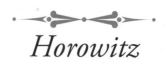

the Creator is said to have "breathed into his nostrils the breath of life; and man became a living soul." (Genesis 2:7) That is, he breathed the math of 8 into him. Element 8 carries the core energy for Divine unity and spiritual transformation along with physical materialization—the miracle of sustaining and creating life as a living soul or spirit.

Thus, you can also think of the term respiration, as re-spiritualizing yourself with every important, virtually sacred, breath.

As previously quoted, Plato's "world soul" emphasized 8 along with the 3, 6, and 9 number set as special in musical-mathematics and creative science.

Although you can't do this with other numbers, if you superimpose the 6 and 9 atop the 3 it looks like an 8. This reflects the symbolism and sacred geometry of these numbers used to manufacture matter.

As you will later learn, the total Matrix of the Creator's math produces the same architecture of twin circles, one atop the other, a figure 8—the double toroid—or double-donut stacked shape of the universe!

So, the Creator is symbolized by 8 that includes in its intelligent design the special number set—3, 6,

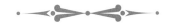
and 9. As you will soon see, these numbers serve as portals to the Divine or spiritual realm that includes the Totality of everything infinitely. That's also why the infinity sign—∞—uses a 90° rotated 8 or two unified circles—∞.

Soon you will learn that at the core of creation are the 528 and 639 Hertz frequencies that resolve to the numbers 6 and 9, respectively. These tones are "MI," for miracles, and "FA," for family. Brought together, these numbers create the symbol "69" widely known as the yin and yang energies of the universe; the male and female counterparts to everything; or the grand polarity of the cosmos.

Merging these polarities as shown in Figure 2 yields the symbol 8 once again, the infinity sign—God's number. 6 and 9 merged also produces the hurricane icon— 6 —indicating the powerful spiraling force of Nature. Likewise, in *Walk on Water*, I reprinted NASA photographs showing the obvious merging of the symbols 6 and 9 to form the spiraling structure of galaxies. Thus, this symbolism and math is being expressed everywhere on Earth as it is in Heaven.

The MIracle 6 number starts at the top and spirals down to rejoin the creative stroke below. Likewise,

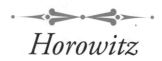

the number 9, indicating completion, spirals up from Earth to the heavens.

These, along with many other revelations, convinced me that math, language, and all of life is based on sacred geometry.

I realized that the encoded electromagnetic frequencies of sound in sacred languages relay spiritual messages between people and between people and God as well.

Add the two most important creative elements—element number one, hydrogen, to element number eight oxygen and you form, according to ancient alchemy and Pythagorean math, 1 plus 8 equals 9—"completion." Indeed, the combination of hydrogen and oxygen makes water which is required to complete creation. The hydroxyl radical OH^- is the chief carrier and balancer of positive and negative charges in electrochemistry and biology. This, more than anything, balances pH fundamental to life.

Recall from the Book of Genesis that in the beginning of creation there was God, the Word, and Water. All three are sacred, yet the masses have forgotten the sanctity of water. Now translate these three words to numbers using the alpha-numeric code

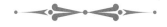

provided and what do you get? God=8, Word=6, and Water=4. Add these numbers to get 18; where 1 + 8 = 9. This is completion once again.

In fact, if you add all the numbers from the alpha-numerics of the English language: 1-9, 1-9, and 1-8, you get 9 again.

Sadly, people have lost knowledge of the sacredness of, besides water, *numbers* and spirituality of language. Re-read *The Word* noting the many references given to water as being essential for creating and sustaining the universe. Even the light came from mathematically energizing the "face of the waters." (Genesis 1:2-3)

As the Bible records, everything was formed from the Creator's word affecting water. Therefore, since math is the Creator's language, if you want to co-create with the Creator using his proven system, you may want to learn to speak His language upon the waters of the world.

There is a Buddhist holyman, Rinpoche, currently traveling around the world blessing water and praying for the lakes, rivers, and oceans. Earth's survival may depend on many more of us doing the same.

You may use your normal language, like English, but sbɾɒwʞɔɒd is best for this Anglo-Saxon "tongue."

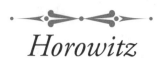

If you desire to be superhuman, expressing your creative self on par with Da Vinci, you must learn to speak the language created by the Supreme Source and Universal Master—the language of ancient mystery-school math.

EXERCISES:

Complete Table 3 below to expand your integration of the English alphabet equivalent of the Pythagorean number system.

1)   Decrypt the pattern hidden within the alphanumerics of English. Go down the list of letters, adding its number to the alpha-numeric result before it. (This is done for the Fibonacci series). List your results in the Total column for a growing total. For example, A=1, B=2, C=3, D=4 and 1+2=3; 3+3=6; 6+4=10 and so on.

2) Find the hidden number pattern 1-3-6-1-6-3-1. Notice also the numbers in the sacred 3, 6, 8, and 9 positions. They yield the 3s, 6s, and 9s.

3) Finally, decipher the complete total value of the whole alphabet to its single digit. Is that completion?

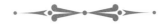

LOVE The Real Da Vinci CODE

Table 3. English Alphabet and Pythagorean Number System.

Number Position	Alpha-numeric Code	Total	Single Digit
1	A 1	1	1
2	B 2	3	3
3	C 3	6	6
4	D 4	10	1
5	E 5	15	6
6	F 6	21	3
7	G 7	28	1
8	H 8	36	**9**
9	I 9	45	**9**
10	J 10	55	1
11	K 11	66	3
12	L 12	78	6
13	M 13	91	1
14	N 14	105	6
15	O 15	120	3
16	P 16	136	1
17	Q 17	153	**9**
18	R 18	171	**9**
19	S 19	190	1
20	T 20	210	3
21	U 21	231	6
22	V 22	253	1
23	W 23	276	6
24	X 24	300	3
25	Y 25	325	1
26	Z 26	351	**9**

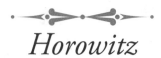

4) Notice the patterns in the multiples of numbers 3, 6 and 9 in Table 4.

a. What is the pattern in the multiples of 3?

b. What is the pattern in the multiples of 6?

c. Is there a pattern in the multiples of 9?

d. If math underlies physics and metaphysics, in fact, everything, does it make sense that everything shares this fundamental creative language?

e. If these patterns present the Creator's creative language, or technology, does it make sense to research and develop this field further with applications of sound and light—mathematical patterns measured in cycles per second—Hz—to address virtually every problem facing humanity today?

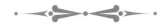

Table 4. Multiples of 3s, 6s, and 9s.

	Multiples of 3	Multiples of 6	Multiples of 9
A 1	1 X 3 = 3	1 X 6 = 6	1 X 9 = 9
B 2	2 X 3 = 6	2 X 6 = 12 – 3	2 X 9 = 18 – 9
C 3	3 X 3 = 9	3 X 6 = 18 – 9	3 X 9 = 27 – 9
D 4	4 X 3 = 12 – 3	4 X 6 = 24 – 6	4 X 9 = 36 – 9
E 5	5 X 3 = 15 – 6	5 X 6 = 30 – 3	5 X 9 = 45 – 9
F 6	6 X 3 = 18 – 9	6 X 6 = 36 – 9	6 X 9 = 54 – 9
G 7	7 X 3 = 21 – 3	7 X 6 = 42 – 6	7 X 9 = 63 – 9
H 8	8 X 3 = 24 – 6	8 X 6 = 48 – 3	8 X 9 = 72 – 9
I 9	9 X 3 = 27 – 9	9 X 6 = 54 – 9	9 X 9 = 81 – 9
J 1	10X3 = 30 – 3	10X6 = 60 – 6	10X9 = 90 – 9
K 2	11X3 = 33 – 6	11X6 = 66 – 3	11X9 = 99 – 9
L 3	12X3 = 36 – 9	12X6 = 72 – 9	12X9 = 108 – 9
M 4	13X3 = 39 – 3	13X6 = 78 – 6	13X9 = 117 – 9
N 5	14X3 = 42 – 6	14X6 = 84 – 3	14X9 = 126 – 9
O 6	15X3 = 45 – 9	15X6 = 90 – 9	15X9 = 135 – 9
P 7	16X3 = 48 – 3	16X6 = 96 – 6	16X9 = 144 – 9
Q 8	17X3 = 51 – 6	17X6 = 102 – 3	17X9 = 153 – 9
R 9	18X3 = 54 – 9	18X6 = 108 – 9	18X9 = 162 – 9
S 1	19X3 = 57 – 3	19X6 = 114 – 6	19X9 = 171 – 9
T 2	20X3 = 60 – 6	20X6 = 120 – 3	20X9 = 180 – 9
U 3	21X3 = 63 – 9	21X6 = 126 – 9	21X9 = 189 – 9
V 4	22X3 = 66 – 3	22X6 = 132 – 6	22X9 = 198 – 9
W 5	23X3 = 69 – 6	23X6 = 138 – 3	23X9 = 207 – 9
X 6	24X3 = 72 – 9	24X6 = 144 – 9	24X9 = 216 – 9
Y 7	25X3 = 75 – 3	25X6 = 150 – 6	25X9 = 225 – 9
Z 8	26X3 = 78 – 6	26X6 = 156 – 3	26X9 = 234 – 9
126	**153**	**153**	**234**
= 9	**= 9**	**= 9**	**= 9**

Notice the multiples of 3 or 6 always yield a 3, 6, or 9.
Multiples of 9 always yield 9—completion.

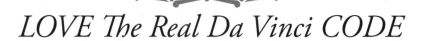

LOVE The Real Da Vinci CODE

Chapter 8
Alpha-Numerics, Creative Spirit, and Completion

According to the Bible, Yah always multiplies or divides and never adds numbers. All multiples of 8 reduced to their Pythagorean single digit integer beginning with 1 X 8 = 8; 2 X 8 = 16 where 1 + 6 = 7; 3 X 8 = 24 where 2 + 4 = 6; and so on as seen in Table 5. The multiples of 8 produce a repeating numerical countdown pattern separated by 9s beginning with 8. That is, 8, 7, 6, 5, 4, 3, 2, 1, **9**, 8, 7, 6, 5, 4, 3, 2, 1, **9**, 8, 7, 6, 5, 4, 3, 2, 1—which corresponded to the alpha-numerics of the English language backwards!

More incredibly, to prove the reversed alpha-numeric perfection of the English language, as shown in Table 5, if you add the alphanumeric equivalents of the English alphabet forwards, to backwards, the sum always results in 9 once again, the number associated with completion.

If you do the same for the Fibonacci series of numbers dismissed as meaningless by Princess Sophie in *The Da Vinci Code*, you get the same 9. Obviously this is a highly significant number which is not meaningless. Especially if you wish to complete Da Vinci's course in creative mathematics for Divine attunement and spiritual development.

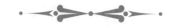

LOVE *The Real Da Vinci* CODE

Number 9 symbolizes spiritual evolution, language completion, and Divine communion—moving up from Earth to the wholeness in Heaven and therein rejoining our Creator in the "Cosmic Circle." That is absolute completion or *complete absolution* in the Catholic sense. This spiraling circle symbolism, and the 9 numbers needed for the grand completion, provides a clue to decrypting the real Da Vinci code.

If there is something spiritually/mathematically sacred about the English language, why is it herein proven alpha-numerically *backwards*?

Here's where the real villains of *The Da Vinci Code* make their debut.

Chapter 9
The Secret Manipulation
of the Masses

Da Vinci lived around the time the German-descended Anglo-Saxon, and later Norman, ruling elite developed and encoded the mathematically/spiritually reversed English language. The King James Bible was written soon after and became the number one work promoting modern English. Obviously, the aforementioned English alphanumeric code, like some of the verse numbering in the Bible, is based on mystery school mathematics. Some historians say Moses†, who wrote the first books of the Bible, and subsequent Levi priests, acquired this creative spiritual technology from the Egyptians and earlier the Babylonians.

As I explained in *Healing Codes for the Biological Apocalypse*, and expanded in *Walk on Water*, my Levitical ancestors translated the Torah into Greek. At that time they encoded the verse numbers in the *Book of Numbers* with the original musical scale.

The esoteric truth about these actions remained hidden from the masses until the publication of *Healing Codes for the Biological Apocalypse* and

---

† See notes for hidden meaning in Moses's name.

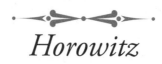

Walk on Water. I concluded the keepers of this sacred knowledge maintained secrecy for two possible reasons: 1) The powerful freeing knowledge of sacred language and mathematics was hidden in an effort to manipulate the unwitting masses by keeping people ignorant, and/or 2) by Divine plan, the world required a maturation period prior to embracing this revelation and mathematical/spiritual emancipation.

In either case, the English language engineers, with certain royal and secret society influence, "confused the tongues" as the Creator had done in Babylonian times.

The Da Vinci Code dimly illuminated this spectre of secret society suppression of critical knowledge along with other politically-explosive manipulations.

Indeed, the suppression of such intelligence, and resulting social ignorance, has mathematically, metaphysically, and spiritually enslaved humanity.

Now, almost everyone is speaking misleading math that is vibrationally dissonant and distancing from their most creative intelligence, spiritual sovereignty, and shared divinity.

You are about to emerge from this darkness, be educated out of ignorance, and help discharge this mass

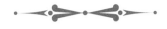

deception. Da Vinci arose to thrive among the world's wealthiest ruling elite including kings, bankers, and popes. If he could use this secret knowledge in this political arena to express super-human genius there's hope for each of us.

It's time to transcend the ruling cryptocracy and the world's overbearing oligarchy.

Table 5. Column Showing Multiples of Eight (8)

Multiple of Eights	Reverse Alphabet	Alphabet w/ Numbers	Sum of Two Alphabet #s
1 X 8 = 0 8 ——— 8 Z		A 1	9
2 X 8 = 1 6 ——— 7 Y		B 2	9
3 X 8 = 2 4 ——— 6 X		C 3	9
4 X 8 = 3 2 ——— 5 W		D 4	9
5 X 8 = 4 0 ——— 4 V		E 5	9
6 X 8 = 4 8 ——— 3 U		F 6	9
7 X 8 = 5 6 ——— 2 T		G 7	9
8 X 8 = 6 4 ——— 1 S		H 8	9
9 X 8 = 7 2 ——— 9 R		I 9	9
10 X 8 = 8 0 ——— 8 Q		J 1	9
11 X 8 = 8 8 ——— 7 P		K 2	9
12 X 8 = 9 6 ——— 6 O		L 3	9
13 X 8 = 104 ——— 5 N		M 4	9
14 X 8 = 112 ——— 4 M		N 5	9
15 X 8 = 120 ——— 3 L		O 6	9
16 X 8 = 128 ——— 2 K		P 7	9
17 X 8 = 136 ——— 1 J		Q 8	9
18 X 8 = 144 ——— 9 I		R 9	9
19 X 8 = 152 ——— 8 H		S 1	9
20 X 8 = 160 ——— 7 G		T 2	9
21 X 8 = 168 ——— 6 F		U 3	9
22 X 8 = 176 ——— 5 E		V 4	9
23 X 8 = 184 ——— 4 D		W 5	9
24 X 8 = 192 ——— 3 C		X 6	9
25 X 8 = 200 ——— 2 B		Y 7	9
26 X 8 = 208 ——— 1 A		Z 8	9

Column of multiples of eights deciphered according to the Pythagorean skein in which all integers are reduced to single digits. Example: 208=2+0+8=10; then 10=1+0=1. This number is associated with the letter A. When A=1 is added to the reverse alphabet letter Z=8, the sum is 9. The number nine (9) implies completion and results everytime the forward and backward English alphanumerics are added together. (See: *Healing Codes for the Biological Apocalypse*, 1999.)

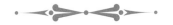
EXERCISES:

1) Using the alpha-numeric code you just learned and integrated in the previous exercise, decipher the math, and single digit (number), for the following words:

6
1
9
2
8

a) Faith : _____ 8 _____

2
9
3
1
b) Trust: 2 _____ 8 _____

7
6
4
c) God: _____ 8 _____

3
9
5
1
2
d) Creator: 8 _____ 8 _____

7
9
6
4
9
4
d) Provider: 8 _____ 8 _____

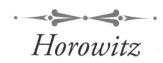
2) Determine the numerical equivalents for the terms listed below.

a) XXX: ___666___ 9

b) FOX: ___666___ 9

c) XOX (As in tic-tac-toe") ___9___

If your results intrigue you, you may appreciate reading the pre-9/11 prophecy, *Death in the Air: Globalism, Terrorism and Toxic Warfare* (www. healthyworlddistributing.com; 1-888-508-4787). You will learn something valuable about the symbolism of the forces of evil profitably operating deceptively throughout the world today.

3) Decipher the infamous Mark-of-the-Beast, "666" to its single digit integer. What is it? State why this is not meaningless? 9

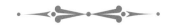

4) Look up Revelation 13:18 in the Bible and write it out below. Consider this as a hint provided about those who control the planet in these years proclaimed the "End Times."

Here is wisdom. Let him hath understanding count the number of the beast. For it is the number of a man and his number is

6 6 6

5) What do you need in order to count a name?

UNDERSTANDING

6) Look up the dimensions of important Bible constructions such as Noah's Ark, Solomon's Temple, and Moses's Tabernacle converting cubits to feet. (1 cubit = 1 foot, 6 inches). What number set is consistently used?

7) In Revelation 14:1, how many people need to sing "a new song" before people stop fighting among themselves? 144,000

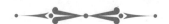

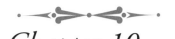

Chapter 10
Why Da Vinci Wrote "Backwords"

Additional clarity as to why Da Vinci wrote "backwords" is available through reverse speech.

In *Healing Codes for the Biological Apocalypse*, I explained why English is a reversal of Hebrew, alphanumerically. Divine communion with the Source of supreme inspiration, I explained, happens every time an Englishman speaks in *reverse*. This revelation should help you view the English-speaking world as spiritually deprived.

"The English language, and speech played backwards, relays truths from the soul," pioneering investigator of "reverse speech," Dr. David John Oates, proclaimed on national radio. He played segments of famous people's speeches in reverse to prove his thesis.

I investigated Dr. Oates's theory and technology to satisfy my curiosity. Based on this study, I concluded, once again, that English is mathematically related to the sacred languages, but electromagnetically or spiritually *backwards*.

This curse of English reflects economics and geopolitics. The British royalty with Anglo-American banking cartel controllers manipulate most

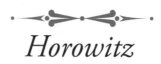
of the world's commerce and geopolitics. This is classically called *neocolonialism* or *globalism.* This English influence is one of the main reasons humanity is morally regressing rather than civilly progressing. Competition versus collaboration, and degenerative consumption rather than sustainable production is their modus operandi.

The globalists' preferred language is English which reads from left to right while sacred languages, such as Hebrew, read from right to left. Why? Because mind control, spiritual warfare, and population manipulation can be best affected by reversing the frequencies of sacred languages. The mathematical polarities of speech are being abused to suppress optimal brain function.

As briefly mentioned, science shows the right hemisphere of your brain is more active spiritually and intuitively. It undoubtedly shares a more peaceful co-existence with your heart. It is generally more receptive, female, and creative. Rational reasoning is processed more by your left hemisphere in your more ego-centric, largely fear-based, thought processing center.

LOVE The Real Da Vinci CODE

Language is similarly divided. In adult brains, language typically activates the left brain. Your right hemisphere, more active in children than adults, engages creative and artistic domains. You might say adults are deprived of natural child-like creative consciousness for this reason. It is the main reversal associated with the "original sin"—the fundamental violation of Divine direction and creative communion for the sake of tempting knowledge. Humanity's left brain speaks while its right heart/brain yearns to sing.

Academically, the left brain serves more scientists; the right side blesses more artists. The two sides are like the "69"—mirror images of one another, or polar opposites. This partly explains the view that "men are from Mars, women are from Venus." It also illuminates the tragedy of a male-dominated patriarchal society that suppresses and abuses women. Women are the most creative and nurturing contributors to civilization. They are obviously being suppressed on a planet governed primarily by patriarchs directing us to the brink of annihilation.

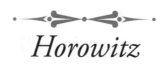

The Law of Love and Prosperity

Male/female harmony must be reestablished to advance common divinity. All relationships are based on faith and trust—mathematical 8s. Male/female relationships are most commonly and heavily challenged by breaches of faith and trust. These occur mostly from communication breakdowns, that is, lost language and missing math.

Misunderstandings, misinterpretations, or failed communications reflect your own deficiencies; that which you haven't owned, integrated, or mastered in your own male/female balanced personality.

The universe is balanced according to mathematical patterns, as you will soon learn. This Law involves cybernetics, that is, feedback loop communications. Stressful relationships do not generally occur by chance. They result from your negligence, or lack of response-ability to feedback you may not wish to receive. Call it justice, judgment, or karma, your problems do not present serendipitously. "Shⵏt happens" for your personal development, clearing of negativity, and heart/mind healing.

In fact, through the mathematical Matrix you will study, you attract precisely what you resist, or reap what you sow, energetically and electromagneti-

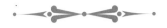
cally. A full understanding of the real Da Vinci code proves this profound understanding very clearly.

In other words, all of your troubles in life stem from "mathematical-masochism." You disable yourself mathematically with self-defeating socially-disruptive communications or bad vibrations. And these choices commonly become habits.

This problem hinges on egocentrism—thinking you are smarter than anything or anyone else. This attitude energetically disrupts your connection to the Matrix, to other people, and to the Most High Source of guidance. This truth is part of the Word and the Law. You can banish your "inner child" this way if you wish, but it will cost you much including love, joy, peace, prosperity and creativity.

Alternatively, like The Renaissance Man who playfully scoffed at the Church's hypocrisy by expressing his creativity through brilliant works of art, you can hold full faith and trust in your connection, communications, and communion within the Matrix.

Rather than living with fear, doubt, anger and disappointment, you hold the power to choose heartfelt Love and confidence in your communion with Yah and others. It's a matter of choice to be led by your heart, and not simply by your head, at every moment.

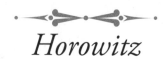

When you lead with your head, you are directed by life experience, past decisions, lessons learned (mostly "the hard way") and commonly fear. Alternatively, when you lead with your heart, you are directed by the vast universe of Love with faith in the unity of humanity living in harmony with Divinity.

As you may instinctively know, and will soon fully grasp, leading with Love relays an extraordinary mathematical frequency that bridges genetic, social, political, economic, and spiritual gaps. You've heard the saying, "Do what you Love and the money will come." So does everything else according to the real Da Vinci code. Heavenly gates open and prosperity pours out when you open your heart to this good vibration.

Much emphasis in the Bible is given to living with a happy heart, especially if you desire to be prosperous in all ways. This point is beautifully addressed by John Hendricks in *Prosperity God's Way*. He makes it clear that "giving and receiving" are energetically the same and interchangeable terms. The phrases "abundant sharing" and "giving and receiving" equally express being in harmony with the principles and truths of God's Word. This is more easily understood with the real Da Vinci code heralding man's com-

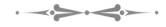

munion with all creation. The mathematical Matrix of the universe, and the cybernetic (feedback) energy dynamics operating in our Kingdom of Heaven, boomerangs your output.

Most importantly, to effectively engage this closed-loop system to reap the greatest rewards, your heart must be fully and *joyfully* engaged. Why? Because this is how the Creator works and how you were created to co-create in joy.

Think about this. You've heard it said, "It is better to give than to receive." The Creator is obviously a great example of this. You are constantly receiving what Yah is giving—the air you breathe, the water you drink, the food for life, and the energy you need to heal and live. This is all given with Love and joy, and in return the Creator receives Love and joy from His relatives who hold faith and trust in the relationship.

Shall we not be imitators of our glorious Creator? If "the Love you take is equal to the Love you make," should we not be pure-hearted givers in every way? "And in this giving," wrote Minister Hendricks, "we will be free and joy-filled, and open floodgates of receiving to ourselves." He concludes, "This is how God set up life, and this is the way to live life."

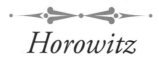

Horowitz

By getting into the groove of abundant, joyful sharing, you engage the Law—the full frequency of giving and receiving. Then our joy-filled Creator, who reads the mathematical vibration of your heart will harmonize with your child-like happiness, and open the floodgates of heaven and pour out abundance for you.

Reversing Wrong Direction

Returning to the topic of reverse speech and the spiritual dynamics of language, children are increasingly being diagnosed with dyslexia, reversing their letters and numbers. This may be occurring more commonly because of an advancing Spiritual Renaissance. In this age of increasing enlightenment, dyslexia may be viewed as nature's attempt to rectify the unnatural retardation imposed by alpha-numerically altered/mathematically-reversed languages.

Think about this. Dyslexic children tend to be more intuitive and artistically creative. They seem to have less trouble expressing their right brains and loving hearts. Yet parents and teachers label them "learning challenged. They are said to need special education, and are required to learn our mathematically-reversed, spiritually-stifling, English language. Ironically, this is called a civilized society, with officials pledging "no child left behind."

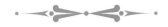

In review and conclusion, when the direction of reading words and articulating them in speech is mathematically reversed, as it is with English, it literally compromises your left-brain/right-brain function, spiritual connection, and optimal genius.

If you were created in the image of the Creator then your lips are also spiritually-creative instruments. This knowledge of language, and its mathematical basis, is necessary for your ascendency to a more sane reality. Live a holistic life in the heavenly domain rather than a fractured co-existence in lunacy. If you use a manner of speaking "taught by the Spirit," as Apostle Paul prescribed in first Corinthians (2:6-16), you will "receive the things from the Spirit of God."

Refined speech and certain tones, sounds, and music, can transmit the Creator's loving vibrations—all math-based expressions of Divinity.

Hold this knowledge dearly and exercise its power. You will use this intelligence to solve the primary problem plaguing humanity since the Tower of Babel—communication. The word itself says it all. It instructs you to *commune* in the Divine community. In this loving family lies your Source of happiness, abundant sustenance, and creative fulfillment.

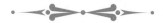

EXERCISES:

1) This week, increasingly bond with others and the Creator in the Spirit of Love. Consciously resolve to connect more sincerely, open-heartedly, more regularly, and joyfully, using communications that reflect your appreciation for the Divine/human family.

This week, have your lips move to express truth with more faith and trust in your loving nature. Then you will commune with the Most High and gain the inspiration and talents of singing from your soul.

2) To regain your essence, wholeness, and heart/mind balance, you simply need to integrate the real Da Vinci code's math which echoes the Creator's language. Write the following simple words backwards to expand your thinking:

a) Dog : _____. Man's best friend.

b) Evil : _____. Draining versus sustaining.

c) Devil : _____ . Adversary outside heaven.

d) No : ___. Limitation versus full operation.

e) Yes : ____. Visualize and speak through the ocean of creation.

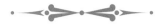

f) AND : _____. Linking everything.

g) From : _____. Means change.

3) From now on, realize the importance of element 8—oxygen, and throw your chest out to expand your lungs and your breath. Lead with your heart, in Love, rather than your head in fear or doubt. Practice righteousness, that is, "right-standingness" by modifying your body posture. Stand up and walk straighter; hold your head up and shoulders back farther, especially if you have forward head posture and/or stooped shoulders. Consciously choose to open your joy-filled loving heart. See if you can realign yourself with the universal flow of mathematical Matrix energy.

4) Read a book or magazine backwards in a mirror for 3, 6, or 9 minutes a day for the next 3, 6 or 9 days. Simply hold the pages in front of a mirror to practice reading backwards. In this way, your brain will engage more balanced data processing, like Da Vinci did, opening more of your creative/intuitive/visionary intelligence.

5) This week, let mathematics speak to you from a higher dimension. For example, many people view 11:11 on a digital clock as a good sign that "all is well in unity with the One."

Other examples abound throughout nature and various cultures. North American natives, for instance, look to numbers in nature, such as a single versus group of crows, wolves, deer, buffalo, etc., to relay messages from The Great Spirit. Sighting a single crow, for example, in native lore, may sound an alert to be on the lookout for danger; whereas two or more crows bade better for the traveler.

This is also academically supported, for example, in Robert Batchelor's Stanford Univ. thesis. Here he explained:

> "[S]cholars of the Renaissance thought of the production of knowledge in terms of reading the book of the world. In a realist sense, God's signs were literally everywhere in nature, so that someone like the famous physician Paracelsus (1493-1541) could argue that "the stars in heaven must be taken together in order that we may read the sentence in the firmament. It is like a letter that has been sent to us from a hundred miles off, and in which the writer's mind speaks to us."

Let Yah speak to you this week through signs and wonders in nature. Paracelsus advocated something similarly in "the doctrine of signatures," in which he claimed sentences made from stars contain divine signatures.

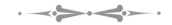

Children, and parents, today envision faces and forms in clouds while in ancient times mystics experienced stars as colorful spheres of sound that communicated God's messages.

According to Batchelor, the Creator's signature is considered key to all of this. "[T]he signature acted as a key to God's great post-Babel cipher. Increasingly, many began to think that the 'key' to the cipher was mathematics."

You will grasp this concept more fully in Chapter 16 where you will see Yah's signature on *everything*.

This week, consider yourself, your communications, and the world around you as encoded mathematics. Recognize this entire system is creative/constructive/productive, loving, and joy-filled by mathematically intelligent design. These recognitions are keys that open the heavenly floodgates to prosperity and more including the "Grand Unification" to be detailed later.

Use the space below to chronicle your experiences this week exercising the aforementioned life-skills. Document your progress and positive results here or in your journal:

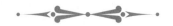

NOTES:

Chapter 11
The Secret Sacred
Spiritual Mechanics of Life

The Holy Spirit, commonly recognized by all religions, uses the dynamics and mechanics of musical–mathematics. This metaphysics inspires life. Biophysics, the energy dynamics fundamental to biology, is a brand of metaphysics. Metaphysical theories and theologies go hand-and-hand with advancing reality theories, mathematics, and the physical sciences. Transcend divisive religious dogma for a moment and cut to the core of Divine creativity.

As I shared in *Walk on Water*, which you are encouraged to read to fully integrate this intelligence, Dr. Hartmut Müller, previously with the Institutes of the Russian Academy of Sciences and the Institute for Applied Mathematics of Leningrad University, now living in the United States, proved that the human spirit, energy field, or biofield, was entrained to a "standing gravitational force field" resonating from the periphery of the cosmos. This field of study is mostly mathematical, sometimes physical, and partly theological, was christened "Biocosmology."

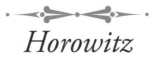

Müller and co-workers showed that your body, like all biology, is mathematically generated piece by piece, or "fractally." Mathematically, you crystallize or fall apart. As an expert in space-time mathematics and physics, Müller compared biological elements to cosmic elements: planets, galaxies and particles in space. Comparing double helix DNA to "the universe as a double helix on the logarithmic line," he concluded, "the genetic code itself is a product of the Global Standing Gravitational Wave = time wave." (See Figures 1 and 2.)

Waves flow according to mathematical law, in fact, *the* Law discussed herein. I have capitalized *Law* so that you will know this is not a lesser law. It is the Supreme Law directing everything.

Müller and colleagues detailed the existence of special "nodes" in this Law he calls the "Global [i.e., universal] Standing Gravitational Wave." All physical elements congeal within this Matrix. From microscopic bacteria and cell parts to macrocosmic celestial bodies and galaxies, all matter crystallizes in special energy zones within this math. He noted that this fractal mathematical-precipitation of matter is based on repeating sequences of the numbers 3, 6, and 9. This set of numbers, along with 8, as you

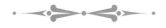
have already learned and will increasingly use, opens the portal to the fourth dimension, future vision, and the spiritual domain. Müller observed experimentally the place from whence everything in the physical universe comes.

Müller wrote of a creationistic transition toward physical precipitation from spiritual ether—from the "unpacked medium" of disorganized or chaotic free energy—the yin, to the "packed cluster medium" of physical objects in space/time—the yang. In scientific terms, you are about to learn the metaphysical secrets of creationistic power; for exercising mathematical heart-mind over matter.

Recall from Chapter 7, you considered the origins of languages and underlying math—the Creator's language that animates your soul, doesn't lie, and knows you intimately. You exercised your right brain by reverse reading and using creative mathematics—especially the 3s, 6s and 9s. Balanced brain function, you recall, was needed for your "Grand Communion."

In the forthcoming exercises, the 3s, 6s, and 9s are shown to reflect each other and intermingle. These numbers, you will see, all derive from the "Grand O" or "Circle of Life" being evenly split.

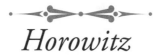

Horowitz

Creation is compelled mathematically quite similarly evolving from initial unity in the whole system to individuality. The initial mathematical clustering or structuring of matter from free flowing randomly-spaced particles in space/time, Müller wrote, was forced by the mathematical Matrix he called the Standing Gravitational Wave. This wave is graphically depicted in Figure 1.

Like waves bouncing off the sides of a swimming pool, the universal wave ricochets in predictable directions. Its bend is predicated on the shifting of numbers 3, 6, and 9. Each place and time the grand wave hits the "light horizon," or virtual cosmic wall, its refraction shifts the Pythagorean trinity—3, 6, and 9 (or energy portal) positions—by a factor of "In(6)."

"In(6)" also relates to the Book of Genesis account of universal creation "in 6 days."

Numbers are sacred symbols—secret messages about the "Cosmic Circle" spiraling to Earth from a spinning Heaven. "As above, so below." According to Müller, all of this occurs along the universe's logarithmic line as determined mathematically and experimentally. Müller and colleagues diagrammed this dynamic in Figure 1.

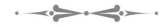
Figure 1 also shows double helix DNA, the sacred spiraling "blueprint of life" that is mathematically, logarithmically, and structurally correlated to the Standing Gravitational Wave.

Can you now understand more clearly why I conclude life spirals down from Heaven to Earth mathematically with DNA being a prime example? This sacred spiral of the creationistic process is generated from patterns of mathematical music. It is likewise capable of recreating life and duplicating itself, just as we now know the Creator does for consciousness and diversity.

Figure 1. Similar Structuring of DNA and Standing Universal Gravity Wave

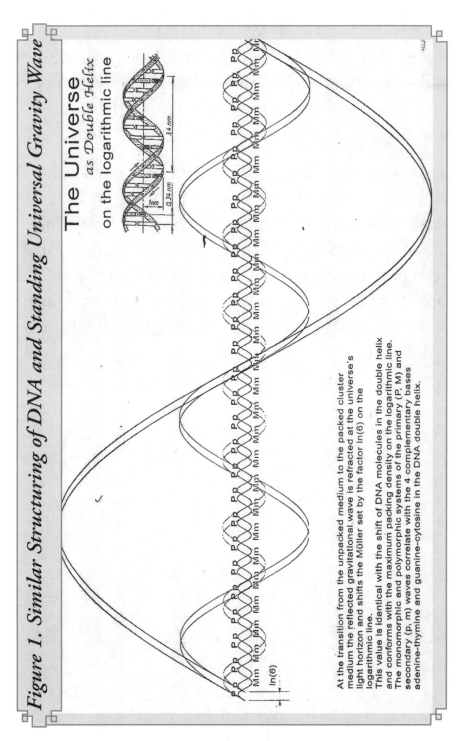

The Universe
as Double Helix
on the logarithmic line

At the transition from the unpacked medium to the packed cluster medium the reflected gravitational wave is refracted at the universe's light horizon and shifts the Müller set by the factor ln(6) on the logarithmic line.

This value is identical with the shift of DNA molecules in the double helix and conforms with the maximum packing density on the logarithmic line. The monomorphic and polymorphic systems of the primary (P, M) and secondary (p, m) waves correlate with the 4 complementary bases adenine-thymine and guanine-cytosine in the DNA double helix.

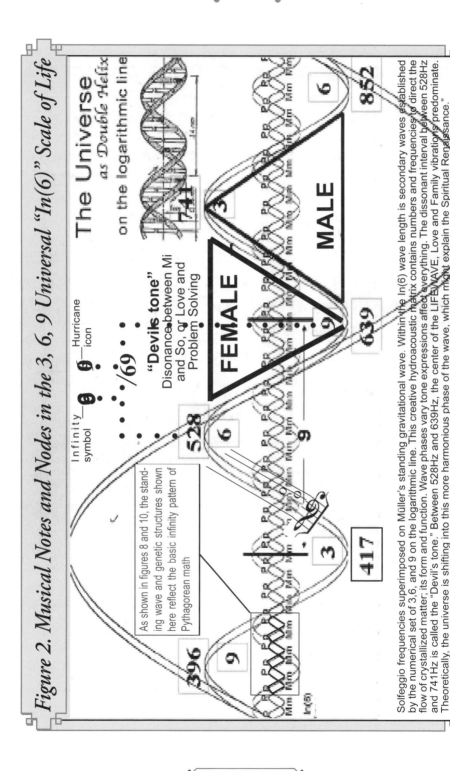

Figure 2. Musical Notes and Nodes in the 3, 6, 9 Universal "In(6)" Scale of Life

The Universe as Double Helix on the logarithmic line

Infinity symbol

Hurricane icon

∞/69

"Devil's tone" Disonance between Mi and So, or Love and Problem Solving

As shown in figures 8 and 10, the standing wave and genetic structures shown here reflect the basic infinity pattern of Pythagorean math

FEMALE

MALE

396   9
528   6
417   3
639   9
741   3
852   6

In(6)

Solfeggio frequencies superimposed on Müller's standing gravitational wave. Within the In(6) wave length is secondary waves established by the numerical set of 3, 6, and 9 on the logarithmic line. This creative hydroacoustic matrix contains numbers and frequencies established the flow of crystalized matter; its form and function. Wave phases vary tone expressions affect everything. The dissonant interval between 528Hz and 741Hz is called the "Devil's tone." Between 528Hz and 639Hz, the center of the LIFE/WAVE, Love and Family vibrations predominate. Theoretically, the universe is shifting into this more harmonious phase of the wave, which might explain the Spiritual Renaissance."

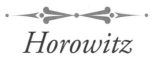
EXERCISES: the origin of number symbols:

1. Complete these exercises in the boxes below.

a. Draw a circle in the first box.
This circle represents everything.

b. Draw "everything" again and a
line cutting the circle in half from far
right to left. This symbol represents
divided unity—man from man; man
from himself; and man from Creator.

c. Imagine the lower half of the circle, the "cup" or "challis," pivoting
in the same plane 180° to the right.
The top half of the circle, the "lid" or
"phallis," stays put. Draw and identify this rudimentary *waveform*.

d, Rotate the lower half of figure b.
45-60° down and to the right. This
rudimentary 9 symbol represents
complete ascendence from Earth to
the Grand Unification.

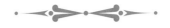
Continue exercise . . .

e. Beginning with Figure b again, pivoting on the right side, move upper and lower halves 90° up and down, respectively, and remove most of the line to form a 3—the trinity of Creator, Created and the Holy Spirit.

f. Rotate the top half of Figure b 45° on its left side. This symbol represents the Divine spiraling down from Heaven to Earth. This symbol represents the numerology of organic chemistry; the basis of life—carbon 6.

g. Now invert both halves of the divided circle symbol you drew in Figure b, and eliminate the center line. This "X" represents the false reversal and division between 2 parts of the whole—the division between male and female parts of equally Divine humanity. This symbol shows the feminine uplifted by the masculine—the challis pivoting on the male phallis symbol.

h. The above "X" symbol, like the circle with a line through it, also represents a divided unity. In this case, man from man; man from himself; and man from Creator.

2. Given the above, can you now see why the numbers 3, 6, and 9 represent a very special set?

3. Study Figure 2, and then:

a. Identify and write in a column the six Hertz frequencies of sound:

_____

_____

_____

_____

_____

_____

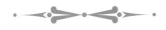
b. Examine the male and female sections of
the Standing Gravitational Wave. Notice the
triangulated energy structure of these segments.
Did you know that the triangle is the "delta"
symbol for change in physics and chemistry?
What, if anything, do you need to change
about your concept of masculinity or feminin-
ity based on this knowledge?

c. Find the musical staff superimposed on
this wave graphic. Can you see how this
mathematical wave may transmit as music?

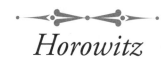

In the last exercises above, ⊖ symbolizes division or the *illusion* of division. It is also depicts a whole note on a musical line. It makes sense that this illusion of a divided whole, a note in music, along with male/female polarity for eternity, was needed to evolve consciousness and self/other recognition. If you were the Creator intent on becoming joyfully self-aware—pleasingly and constructively self-conscious—you too would need to create the illusion of division wouldn't you? Then you would need a code composed of symbols or signals that describe all parts of your whole, would you not?

Does the 1-9 numbering system provide this?

Indeed it does. Everything evolves from the whole or Holy unity symbolized by the circle. The false division, a straight line, represents the shortest distance beween two points—Yah and man. All other numbers derive from this illusion of division as shown in the symbols you just drew.

Besides knowing you derive your existence from math, or Yah's language, an additional way to become self aware, or conscious about yourself, is to reflect from a second vantage point—through another person's eyes or looking at your reflection in a mirror. Distinguishing positive from negative, right from left, male from female, develops this advantage

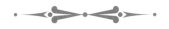

or vantage point. After all, if everything was always positive, then negative would disappear (putting a lot of profiteers out of business). This understanding is basic to metaphysics 101.

So the Creator's only intelligent choice was to divide his creative Self into positive and negative, plus or minus, male versus female, yin and yang, etc. Only then could Yah remain joyfully and universally Self-conscious.

This is why wise men throughout the ages have always prescribed self knowledge. "Know thyself!" Because if you maintained optimal self-knowledge as Yah knows Himself, you would be positively and infinitely self-conscious at the level of the grand mathematical Matrix. That is, with enlightened awareness you would playfully commune, sing and dance, with the musical–mathematical Oneness of space/time and the cosmic community. This would place you home in the Kingdom of Heaven, appreciating the surrounding beauty being created every moment; with none of the mad mentality.

In essence, you'd be free to flow in your life with the unified field of creative possibilities—free to choose your life and be at cause instead of being a victim of negative circumstances.

LOVE *The Real Da Vinci* CODE

If, and when, you created anything negative in your life you would know you did so. You would immediately forgive yourself for all self-inflicted injury you chose. Any other choice would be nonsensical or plainly insane.

So it's your choice to acquire a good life versus traumatic, be productive rather than wasteful, and pleased versus pained. Whatever you choose, you do so based on the aforementioned math.

Therefore, the first smart decision you need to make is whether you choose to acquire a joyful relationship with the math Maker by communing in the Matrix. You will learn more about this Matrix in the coming pages.

Finally, this information further helps explain why "men are from Mars, and women are from Venus." The opposite sexes require one another to model and mirror their missing virtues. You need the opposite sex to develop self-consciousness; to see yourself in the mirror of love versus fear. Isn't that a fact, albeit frustrating for most people?

How much longer must you suffer in your relationships before realizing you're choosing madness over bliss? Why not choose to attract allies not adversaries? We evolved from the Dark Ages. People need to view these "wholes" in their mirrors. It's time to transform ourselves in the image of Yah.

Chapter 12
Genetically Speaking Truth

Genetics, like all matter, represents the physical crystallization of energized math. The intelligence for genetic construction flows freely and lawfully from the Matrix with mathematical precision like a broadcasting station transmits a radio or television signal. Your stream of consciousness or enlighten- ment flows the same way with frequencies of sound (Hz) and wavelengths of light (nm) called phonons and photons, respectively. The sacred resonating geometry of DNA, and its related force-fields, af- fecting and connecting you with everything in the universe, I documented in detail in *DNA: Pirates of the Sacred Spiral.*

A consensus of Bible scholars and space/time physi- cists is now forming. Astrophysicists agree that the mathematics of sound affects water, both present throughout space. In fact, sound and water are two fundamental requirements for the creation of mat- ter. This combination of musical-mathematics af- fecting water miraculously manifests everything.

Most fascinating to me is that the In(6) wave phase, or complete sine wave cycle of universal creation, corresponds to the mathematics and harmonics of

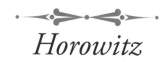

the original Solfeggio musical scale. These musical tones—mathematical frequencies—were encoded by my Levitical ancestors in the Bible's Book of Numbers. In the book, *Healing Codes for the Biological Apocalypse*, these creative frequencies were revealed for the first time in nearly 3,000 years. This revelation has come to benefit humanity. As will be shown shortly, this musical-mathematics, sung from the depths of the cosmic ocean, creates the Standing Gravitational Wave, Love, and all matter. You included!

The book *Walk on Water* explains how and why this ancient musical scale, and advancing new music based on it, will be used to affect a complete turnaround in the governing versus stewarding of our planet. In Christian theology, this is prophesied with the gathering of "New Song" singers, 144,000—1+4+4=9—completion! (Rev. 14:1.)

This knowledge predicts a paradigm shift from our current predominating physical focus, linear intellect, fear-based consciousness, and devilish addictions, to a spiritual transcendence of deficiencies, imbalances, and inadequacies. You are being given a choice to evolve with unlimited creative capacity, including miraculous material manifestations, to revolutionize civilization. All of this is what Da

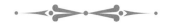

LOVE The Real Da Vinci CODE

Vinci foresaw and heralded with his works of art and science, particularly The Vitruvian Man.

EXERCISES:

If the Creator of life used math as His/Her creative technology, you would expect to see evidence of this math in the code for life called DNA. These exercises provide this proof as to why the basic building block of life—genetics—is encoded in the shape of a spiraling double helix.

1. Using the circle provided in the space below, write the numbers 1 - 9 isometrically, that is, evenly spaced, next to and outside your circle beginning at the top with 9. Your final numbered circle should be like the one shown in Figure 8. But don't fill in the design yet.

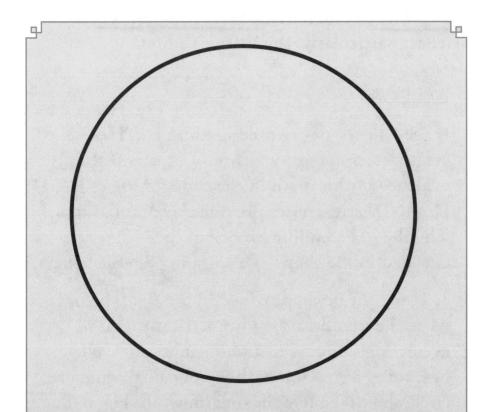

2. Next, fill in the blanks in the number series below to determine the secret mathematical sequence underlying the code for life. Beginning with the number one, double each number and decipher each number down to the Pythagorian single digit integer. (Example: 2x8 = 16, where 1+6=7.)

1, 2, 4, ___, 7, ___, 1, ___, 4, ___, 7, 5, ___, 2, ___, ___, 7, ___.

3. Now, using the circle you numbered, connect the numbers from the code of life you just identified in the order of their pattern. Your final drawing should be similar to Figure 8.

4. This number sequence continues to infinity and is called the "infinity pattern." Can you see the double winged infinity pattern shape created by this mathematical sequence? Yes or No?

Can you see the resemblance of the double-winged infinity pattern you drew and each segment of DNA in Figure 10.

5. Can you see the absence of the 3s, 6s and 9s in this infinity pattern? Yes or No?

6. On the circle, connect the 3, 6, and 9. Can you see this set of numbers maintains a unique triangular geometry or trinity pattern, distinct from the infinity pattern? Yes or No?

7. The 3s, 6s, and 9s, and their triangularity in space/time, theoretically opens portals or doorways to higher dimensions, higher consciousness, or holy spiritual domains from whence Divine creative energies can be relied upon to flow. Matter precipitates or manifests from spirit through this portal system.

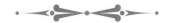

8. In *Walk on Water* and *DNA: Pirates of the Sacred Spiral*, I proposed that DNA operates like an antennae to Yah. Can you now see how this truth is based on simple mathematics?

9. This week, as you travel, see if you can determine the geometry of the antennae used to broadcast cell phone communications. What is this structure? Why do you think this structure is used for wireless communications more than any other geometric form?

10. Through Philomath—the Love of learning and applying this Matrix math—can you now comprehend how Da Vinci might have been able to connect with a Divine Source of intelligence—mathematically-charged pure creativity?

Answer "Yes" to all of the above questions before proceeding, since these simple understandings are fundamental to your ability to commune (or entrain), like Da Vinci, with the Heavenly Matrix.

Chapter 13
Monochord Mathematics
and the Macro/Microcosm

According to historians, a musical instrument called the *monochord* played a harmonious role in architecture, politics, and philosophies upon which civilizations have been built including our own. Among his dying words, Pythagoras is reported to have recommended monochord instruction to his disciples. Plato is believed to have done the same in his addendum to his Laws, called the *Epinomis*. This instrument, it is said, holds the keys to understanding the workings of the universe.

The title, *Epinomis*, references the most important or highest value numbers. It is the only work in the entire body of Plato's productions that specifically addresses the importance of harmonic mathematics and mathematical ratios.

According to expert Graham Pont, "the harmonic analogia or tuning module of 6:8::9:12 [Epinomis 991a-b]," is centrally important. "Analogia means, '*equality of ratios*' or 'proportion,'" The word shares similar roots with the terms analysis, logic, and analogy or similarity. Pont wrote, "the analogia is the module or system of whole-number ratios that gives

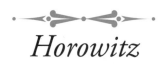

the 'divisions of the monochord,' the precise points at which the vibrating string can be stopped with a movable bridge, to sound the 'fixed' or fundamental intervals of the musical scale, the octave (2:1); the fifth (3:2); the fourth (3:4); and the major tone (8:9). [Once again, t]he integers 6, 8, 9, and 12 are the smallest whole numbers with which the symmetrical system of interlocking ratios—the natural framework of the ancient and modern diatonic scales—can be expressed." The exercise you completed in the last section reflects this "symmetrical system of interlocking ratios."

As already mentioned, the whole note in music is written as an oval. It looks like a zero on its side. When in the middle of a line of music it looks just like a circle cut in half like the drawing you created in Chapter 11, Exercise 1b. To reiterate, this symbol obviously gave rise to the 3, 6, 8, and 9 set of special creative numbers. The oval or circle also relayed the concept that the universe is composed of two equal and opposite parts—an "equality of [male and female] interlocking ratios." This was symbolized by the phallus and challis halves of the equally-divided circle.

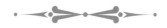

Symbolically then, the zero (0) cut in half, like the eight (8), relays the concept of there always being two halves to one wholeness or unity. The cut, or middle dividing line, (like Ø) represents the fact that opposites are really part of the same circle.

This circle represents the alpha and the omega (the beginning and the end) that our Creator characterizes Himself as being to Moses in the *Book of Exodus*. In a circle, the beginning is also the end. This relates energetically to the concept mentioned in Chapter 3 that giving, or tithing, is the same as receiving. The seeming opposites are interdependent, operating cybernetically, or energetically looped, by a spinning circular monochord.

Here is another way of contemplating this universal freeing truth. Polarity exists for everything, and everything and nothing are really the same. How so?

If you were everything, like the Creator that manifests into all creation, then there would be nothing else. So everything and nothing are like opposite sides of the same coin. If one side disappears so must the other. Likewise, if one side manifests, so must the other.

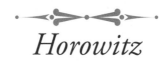

The aforementioned duality and polarity relates to the circular monochord as well. This circular instrument, according to authorities, played into existence the basis for all experience and existence.

In *The Pythagorean Plato* (1978) Ernest McClain discusses the fundamentals of tuning and features the circular application of the monochord string. I suggest you consider this along with the importance of tuning into the "Circle of Life." If you were to commune with the frequencies of the monochord, how might this affect your health, well-being, and prosperity?

"As above so below." If the cosmos springs from a sacred circle of sound, the monochord, Heaven must present musically to Earthlings.

McClain explained that the monochord tones can be graphed geometrically, or circularly. This idea of graphing sound, laying specific tones out on a circular line, is precisely what I did when I first conceived of the "Perfect Circle of Sound."

The implications of this knowledge are broadly transformational. Taken to the next level, McClain's text examined seven of Plato's numerical allegories as they relate to his theories of music underlying politics, empowered governors, and governments. It has

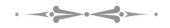

LOVE The Real Da Vinci CODE

been reported that the governmental constitutions of Athens, Callipolis, Atlantis, and Magnesia, according to McClain, corresponded to four different tuning systems, or musical temperaments.

This may seem irrelevant, but I assure you it's important if we wish to transform global politics and disharmonious governments into something more sensible.

Linking musical-mathematics to civilizations past and present, Pont examined the "Predecessors of Pythagoras" in relation to architecture, especially focused on temple art. He noted "their connection with science and music." In the "grandest monuments that man has built in imitation of the heavenly order," monochord musical-mathematics is apparent.

Joseph Campbell, a leading metaphysical historian, reviewed five millennia of cultural development. He showed temple designs consistently included traditional mandalas of the circle and square—ancient symbols of Heaven and Earth. This graphic encryption of the ancient monochord is likewise displayed in many of the world's financial and governing capitals, including London, Paris and Washington, D.C. Da Vinci's Vitruvian Man also displays this as will be analyzed later.

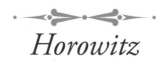
Additional evidence of the importance and application of this circular geometry in government and finance is found in the research of Michael Mackay, an independent investigator.

Figure 3 provides a crude view of planet Earth seen from outer space above the North Pole. Mackay graphed the energy grid, called Lay lines, throughout the Northern hemisphere. Astonishingly, the Western world's major financial and governing capitals including London, Paris, Rome, Cairo/Jerusalem, New York, Boston, Philadelphia, Washington D.C., and Atlanta share nearly the same Lay line! This is obviously a monochord, harmonically resonating in each precise location, to express optimal economic and political clout and generate massive wealth for the keepers of this secret sacred creative knowledge.

Now you can begin to fathom the ramifications of this discovery, its political implications, and the revolutionary opportunity we hold to level the playing field for creative control over planet Earth, including financial control.

Near the beginning of this book, I informed you this knowledge demands a high level of responsibility. I said it would challenge your personal collaborative integrity. Now that you have a more complete pic-

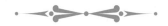

ture, are you now more interested in teaming up to advance our planet's redirection? It does not appear to be an intelligent option to remain ignorant, fearful, and thus part of the planet's main problem—ignorance of *this* truth that can set everyone free.

Use Da Vinci as your model. What did he do with his knowledge? He advanced a new view of the world. He shared his knowledge and creativity to the best of his ability, and his work has lasted the test of time.

You are about to receive substantial proof that the real Da Vinci code is your ticket to freedom—the master method for recreating yourself and our planet. Drawing on the image of Yah, this path accords with the one Law, one Word, and only one way that makes rational sense. It offers a proven way to command the forces of nature to serve constructively, lovingly, and sustainably, rather than destructively, fearfully, and terminally. This option respects, rather than abuses, the mathematical Matrix and musical monochord.

The potential offered here, as well as the plan, is depicted and encrypted in Leonardo's Vitruvian Man. The drawing is a cryptograph—a secret map of the monochord for biological tuning and spiritual awakening. It incorporates both circle and square,

Figure 3. Mackay's Research on Global Grid Showing Major Financial and Global Geopolitical Power Centers

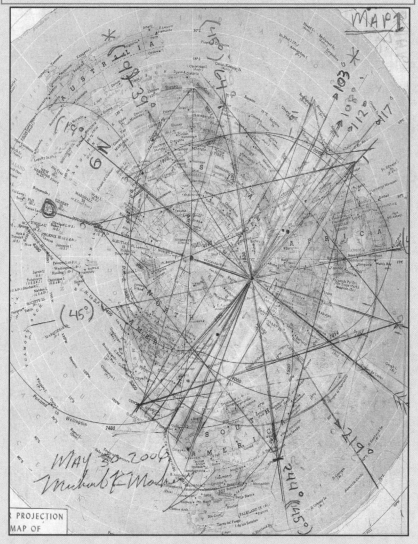

Energy grid, called Lay lines, throughout the Northern hemisphere is graphed showing the Western world's major financial and governing capitals including London, Paris, Rome, Cairo/Jerusalem, New York, Boston, Philadelphia, Washington D.C., and Atlanta share nearly the same Lay line! This monochord apparently resonates each precise harmonic location to express optimal economic and political power.

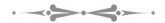

Figure 4. Earth's Sacred Geometric Grid and the Expression of Geopolitical Power & Economic Control

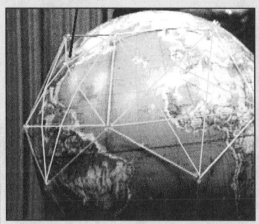

Because if its self-symmetry and use of the Golden Proportion, as shown in Figure 14 the pentagram contains within itself the seed of its own replication in progressively smaller or larger scales. Today this is called fractal geometry. It is the governing template of nature that is also expressed economically and geopolitically throughout the world.

Historically, archaeologists discovered pentagrams on Mesopotamian potsherds dating back to 3500 BC. Pentagrams appear in art from ancient Egypt, Greece, and Rome. Reference to the pentagram in Christian writings stems from Hildegard of Bingen. The twelfth century Benedictine nun perceived the pentagram, as Da Vinci did in creating The Vitruvian Man, as the central symbol of the micro/ macrocosm, reflecting Earth in the Divine plan according to the Creator's image. Hildegard wrote the pentagram metaphorically represented human nature with five obvious senses – sight, smell, 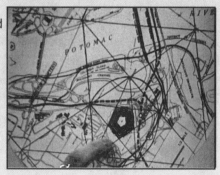 taste, touch, and hearing; and five extremities – two ams, two legs, and a head. And, because humans were made in the Creator's image, she viewed the pentagram as a sacred geometric godly symbol. Christians later saw the pentagram as depicting the five wounds of Christ and, because of this, the symbol was believed to guard against evil. Earlier, Hebrew scholars linked the Pentateuch, the first five books of the Bible, to the pentagram.

Geopolitically, as shown above, the planet's Lay lines provide an energetic template within which pentagonal fractals, like puzzle pieces, fit

Continued on next page.

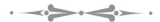

Figure 4 continued . . .

together to complete the global grid. Here, a finger points to the precise construction, and orientation, of America's "Pentagon"—the center of the world's military might—in Washington DC as fitting the global grid. The Pentagon's pentagonal grid points precisely to the White House.

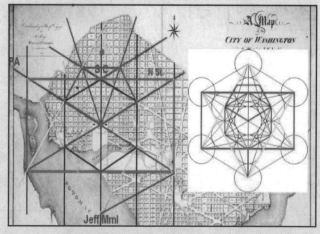

One anoynymous analyst of this sacred pentagon grid wrote his concerns about this extension of Washington's pentagon grid and White House "onto the dodeca Planet." He wrote of troubling geomantic magnetic forces that could affect emotions and mental functions. He predicted if left unchecked, this power would control the geomantic "body politic."

Numerous investigators have critically analyzed the lay-of-the-land and architecture in America's capitol. It is strikingly Masonic in design including the precise locations of Washington's famous monuments. The city's heredity interweaves little known European and Native American

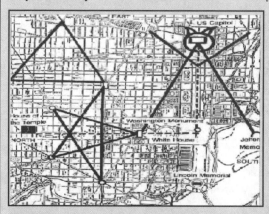

esoterics, wisdom, and traditions. The Capitol Mall design, for instance, incorporates a great circle with a cross representing more than the four elements. The Capitol Building, the White House, the Lincoln Memorial, the Washington Monument, and other featured monuments are laid out like an "X".

These graphics prove secret planners used Metatron's cube (shown top right), containing the "Tree of Life," to design D.C. with 11 of 13 major monuments falling precisely on the global grid.

See: http://soulinvitation.com/WASHINGT/dcfrac.htm and
http://www.geocities.com/jussaymoe/dc_symbolism/index.htm

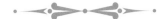

Figure 5. Currency For Controlling Power & People

Shown here is some of the unpublished research of Michael Mackay, a veteran cryptologist decoding the sacred seal and imagery of American currency and coins. His work demonstrates the precise application of sacred knowledge herein explained pertaining to the mathematics of creativity and the alpha-numerics of language. Few people realize that Masonic symbols and architectures adorn every angle of American currency, front and back. Mackay's example is the back side of the common quarter. It is alpha-numerically and geometrically decrypted. Notice the eagle—a Roman symbol for strength in the feminine principle of the pentagram. Its head is slightly off center as are the words above its wings. This is done to encode the double pentagon of the two-headed eagle crest of Russia–Roman royalty into the American coin with the

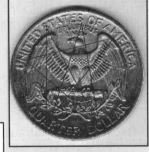

points spelling "MASON." Its slight left leaning implies political orientation. Mackay deciphered this by using the alpha-numeric code revealed herein. This anagram yields the numbers 18 or 81. Confirm this for yourself. This quarter design geometrically emulates the precise angles (degrees) of the Knights Templar shield with two swords as shown lower-right. The swords create

a cross inside the Knights' Black Cross Pattée. (The Knights were "Double Crossed" by the Catholic Church.) These crosses also symbolize the union of Divine male and female elements in all directions. The double pentagram anagram shown above also decrypts to the "Son o[f] man (Christ) Nos (knows)." The Latin word anagram in the Templar shield also codes for Genesis and renewal through knowledge of Judeo-Christian faith. For more on Mackay's research see References & Notes at the end of this book.

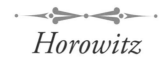

bridging Heaven and Earth, through the monochord nodes—the notes of the "Perfect Circle of Sound."

This is the only reasonable analysis of this art as per Da Vinci's, and his mentors', writings and these recent revelations. This art offers Da Vinci's technical direction for advancing The Universal Man. By understanding, honoring, and applying this knowledge, access to the Matrix — the Kingdom of Heaven— is available to you and everyone called to gather more meaning in life.

The Matrix is the secret sacred musical-mathematics of universal construction. The monochord plays the music of the Matrix. The Matrix is reflected in the Lay lines of this planet, our architecture; even our currency. Its tonal mechanics and geometrics will be revealed to you. By helping to spread this knowledge the world may regain its Divinity.

Look at how other civilizations and scholars applied this knowledge to spark your future vision.

Joseph Campbell observed that the hieroglyphic for ancient Egyptian towns was a St. Andrew's cross inscribed in a circle. It has arms, like Da Vinci's Vitruvian Man, pointing outward "to the minor directions." Campbell discussed the relevance of these symbols to the rise of the ancient city-state 3500-2500BC:

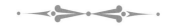

LOVE *The Real Da Vinci* CODE

...The whole city now (not simply the temple area) is conceived as an imitation on earth of the celestial order -- a sociological middle cosmos, or mesocosm, between the macrocosm of the universe and the microcosm of the individual, making visible their essential form: with the king in the center (either as sun or as moon, according to the local cult) and an organization of the walled city, in the manner of a mandala, about the central sanctum of the palace and the ziggurat; and with a mathematically structured calendar, furthermore, to regulate the seasons of the city's life according to the passages of the sun and moon among the stars; as well as a highly developed system of ritual arts, including an art of rendering audible to human ears the harmony of the visible celestial spheres. It is at this moment that the art of writing first appears in the world...[Campbell 1990, 151-2; Pont, 2004]

Can you imagine living during the time Campbell described? Consider yourself at the forefront of this prompt transformation in communications—written works and words created for the first time from sacred sounds, symbols, and math. Imagine serving a similar evolutionary purpose today with this new knowledge you are gaining. Can you grasp this opportunity for creative innovation? Are you ready, willing, and able to make a social contribution for civilization's Divine resurrection?

Graham Pont, in his book *Transforming Total Art*, similarly summarized these implications for evolving humanity. These "connections with the old tradition," he said, are all "symptomatic of a new era in

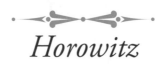
the history of thought when mechanistic and reductionist paradigms are giving way to a holistic and organic world-view. This emergent rationality is fundamentally ecological and its impact is being felt from metaphysics to everyday manners. The new paradigms of the Age of Ecology are already transforming the professions, sciences, arts, academic disciplines, and human enterprises generally—from the minute study of bird-song and insect music to the utopian vision of planet Earth designed and managed as a single, organic Gesamtkunstwerk (i.e., community enterprise).[Pont 1997]

"Decades ago, de Chardin realized that central to this new understanding of the world is the concept of the 'Biosphere,' which is the very antithesis of Newton's mechanistic universe.[Teilhard de Chardin 1955] Likewise, the English geneticist Rupert Sheldrake presented his notion of Nature occurring as a result of 'morphic resonance.'"

Based on the Pythagorean tradition, the real Da Vinci code revealed here manifests like "frozen music" into the architecture of nature, politics and civilization.

"How else are we to explain Vitruvius's frequent references to music?" Pont rhetorically asked. "If the ancient priests, sages, and philosophers were able to discern musical proportions in the heavenly systems,

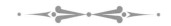
would they not have naturally encoded them in their earthly imitations—just as their predecessors imitated the dance of the stars?"

Answering his own question, Pont concluded, "a discordance between the macrocosm and the microcosm seems unthinkable."[Pont 2004]

EXERCISES:

1) Think of three projects that will bring you additional wealth that integrate this knowledge.

2) If you can't think of three, then practice communing in the Matrix with your most trusted spiritual guide(s). With heartfelt loving intent decree or claim your possession of how you can use this new knowledge for profitable human service without fear or attachment to any outcome. In other words, shut off your head and open your heart-mind.

3) Continue exercising your heart-mind by recalling the symbolism presented in the 3s, 6s, 8s, and 9s. Daily contemplate the polarity/unity duality in: addresses, license plates, hotel room numbers, prices of items, etc. Recall often the hidden meanings of mathematical symbols; particularly the zero.

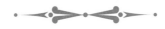

Remember, these seemingly meaningless exercises actually serve to connect your heart-mind to the ancient symbols and freeing truths that reinforce your connection to the Matrix. This will help you develop right-brain consciousness. Increasingly, you will be thinking with your heart as your head gets a deserved vacation.

4) What are your repeating numbers. List one or more numbers you see most often that may represent a sign, signal, symbol, or message from your spiritual guide(s) or Creator.

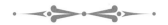

Chapter 14
Da Vinci's Time Travel Technology

Truth has a way of surfacing or resurging. I have seen this time and time again during my past quarter-century as a health science investigator

On the other hand, I have observed numerous times astonishing scientific revelations and major break-throughs disappeared from the public's view, almost immediately, lost to obscurity. I do not perceive this as idiosyncratic, or simply chance. There are methods of mass-mediated mind-control being used. Left-brains, mind-egos, are being manipulated for politics and profits. These methods of psychological warfare stifle the heart-mind. Counter-intelligence propaganda and disinformation condemns humanity to ignorance and virtual slavery. Half truths, if not complete lies, are told for optimal oligarchy control of geopolitics and global economics.

The book and movie, *The Da Vinci Code*, is a prime example of this subtle art of deception. The title begs the question, "Where is the code in *The Da Vinci Code*?" The ploy leaves people ignorant and divided. Is this result accidental in a media-manipulated world wherein global industrialists strive for this "divide-and-conquer" outcome? Popular dependence on prod-ucts such as fuel and drugs is best accomplished with half truths and complete lies.

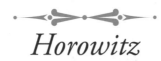

Horowitz

I am not saying Dan Brown is guilty of anything except writing an interesting and controversial novel. The same for Ron Howard and his film. If their prime purpose was to draw popular attention to Da Vinci's esoteric art and secret society geopolitics then they were successful. Far more is needed, however, to raise awareness that Da Vinci's genius and artistic expressions involved a secret code essential for humanity's emancipation from geopolitical manipulations and spiritual damnation.

The mass media should have an important educational role to play. This is true worldwide and clearly expressed in America's *Declaration of Independence* and *U.S. Constitution*. To maintain a balance of powers over unruly governments now heavily influenced by multi-national corporations, it is the media's responsibility, along with every persons', to protest and defend against socially-destructive abuses of power including a deceptive press.

One chief method of public deception is to kill a legitimate story by coverage in one or more of the supermarket tabloids. Mixed among these publications' facts are obvious absurdities. The ridiculous sensationalism functions to discredit reputable books, films, scientists and research discoveries that might otherwise establish widespread publicity, credibility and thus contribute greatly to educate society. Such is the case regarding Leonardo da Vinci's alleged capacity to time travel.

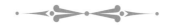

LOVE *The Real Da Vinci* CODE

As reported in *The Sun*, July 17, 2006, "Da Vinci was a time traveler." Allegedly, following 15 years of studying Da Vinci's notebooks, Vatican archivist Monsignor Bruno Pantaleone, reported on Da Vinci's capacity to "describe life in the 20th century in great detail." He concluded Da Vinci's skill was due to the fact that "he had seen it with his own eyes."

The Sun noted that one of Da Vinci's notebooks held scientific information about a method for reversing the flow of time. "Following this is a list of inventions underneath the heading: 'Useful for the advancement of this species, culled from their own future time-line in accordance with our standard protocols.'"

Da Vinci's "descriptions of twentieth century life," included ". . . the development of antibiotics, the Holocaust, the atomic bombing of Japan and the American political system, with special mention of Nixon's resignation . . . ," the Sun mentioned.

Pantaleone analyzed Da Vinci's notebooks for "clues to two remaining mysteries: what method Leonardo da Vinci used to travel through time, and where he came from originally. Neither certainty was determined.

"'The level of knowledge, insight and compassion contained in his notebooks are beyond human,' Pantaleone declare[d]. 'Perhaps, when he refers to 'our standard protocols,' it means that he was from an

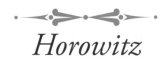
advanced alien race watching over us, or perhaps he was simply a miraculous genius sent by . . . God."

A third possibility, not mentioned, is that the "standard protocols" pertain to the controversial Protocols of the Elders of Sion. [See: *Healing Codes for the Biological Apocalypse*, 1999] The Protocols are believed to have been leaked by one or more leaders of the House of Rothschild in the Prieure du Sion. This later organization is credited in the introduction to *The Da Vinci Code* as implicated in the world's ongoing turmoil along with the radical Catholic sect Opis Dei.

Whether this report, or Da Vinci's ability to time-travel, is factual or not, The Renaissance Man's ability, standard protocol, and technology for prophetic vision would have depended on the science advanced by Müller in time/space physics, and its underlying musical-mathematics. Given that Da Vinci was a master of polyhistor and philomath, Pantaleone's thesis is temptingly credible.

Consciousness is humanity's greatest frontier. Given substantial evidence of intuition, premonition, extrasensory perception, and "remote viewing," it is highly likely that Da Vinci was not in a space-vehicle when he observed with his own eyes the future. Proper balanced brain function, placid cognition, and mathematical-Matrix-connection best explains Da Vinci's astonishing future-vision and prophetic accomplishments.

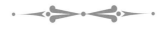

LOVE The Real Da Vinci CODE

I have added these exercises for you to realize that anything and everything is possible with the actual mathematical code Da Vinci used. Though this has been historically suppressed, it is presented below for your consideration, integration, personal mastery, and planetary contribution.

EXERCISES:

1) Fill in the following blanks to complete the mathematics (and Hertz frequencies of sound) that comprise the "Perfect Circle of Sound" and Heavenly Matrix. To do this, simply complete the sequence of numbers placed in the hundreds, tens and ones places.

1 7 4, 2 8 5, __ 9 __, 4 __ __, __ 2 __, 6 __ __, 7 __ 1, 8 __ __, 9 6 3.

2) Lay these numbers out isometrically, that is, evenly spaced, on the circle provided on the next page. Start at the top with the number 396 (the first tone of the ancient scale).

Finally, connect the triads, that is, draw straight lines between the three similar numbers to form the sacred geometrics of this two dimensional "Perfect Circle of Sound."

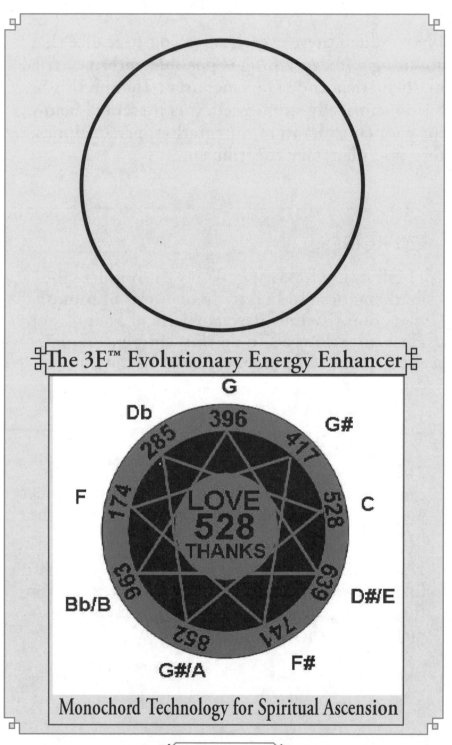

The 3E™ Evolutionary Energy Enhancer

Monochord Technology for Spiritual Ascension

Chapter 15
Grasping This Opportunity

In *Walk on Water*, I explained the power of sound (including words and music) to create everything. My reason for suggesting you study this is the same as what Jesus (actual Hebrew name is YahShuah) intended when he said, "But seek ye first the Kingdom of God, and His righteousness; and all these things shall be added unto you." If you want to have an abundant and fruitful life you will heed this counsel.

Communing with the Matrix is akin to entering the Kingdom of Heaven where everything is ordered here according to the Creator's mathematical Law. Standing *right* in this, that is righteousness, creates miraculous manifestations since there is "nothing missing or broken in the Kingdom of Heaven." Here, everything is possible and readily provided including great wisdom, wealth, creative talents, and health.

This dynamic human ability of communion with the Divine Matrix, through and from which the Holy Spirit flows, is also fundamental to baptisms. Water, after all, is now widely known to be a carrier of consciousness thanks to repeated demonstrations and research by Dr. Masaru Emoto. As viewed on the website www.3epower.us, in figures 15–17, and

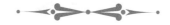

LOVE *The Real Da Vinci* CODE

in Dr. Emoto's amazing books, (See: www.healthy-worlddistributing. com) water molecules comprise a creative fluid that responds to positive prayers and loving intent. *Water is brewing with creative, sustaining, and rejuvenating power.*

If you don't believe this, simply consider some facts: Why do you feel so much better after bathing, showering, or a swim in the ocean? The fact is, you are being spiritually-energized, by immersion in water because the sacred geometry of this liquid energetically relays the musical-mathematics you are learning here—nature's harmonics and balance.

Since you are mostly water, and so is the universe, you resonate with the larger body of water. The universe carries hidden "messages from water," especially Love. Its awesome force compels entrainment with this Law. Thus, you feel refreshed and spiritually blessed from water immersions.

This sacred, secreted, creative knowledge, along with the following mathematical revelations, will trigger your inspirational ideas and technological inventions as you increasingly integrate these symbols, numbers, and fundamental truths. Thus, as a philomath student you can master polymath like Da Vinci.

Chapter 16
The Mathematical Matrix
of the Universe

Central to this amazing opportunity for expanding your creativity is the breakthrough in mathematical understanding conceived by Marko Rodin. The mathematical dynamics of the universe, musically unfolding within a sea of possibilities set in motion by a Standing Gravitational Wave, can be most readily appreciated by studying the wave-like patterns in Rodin's math as shown in figures 6-8.

Rodin's math proves the nine core creative frequencies of the universe. Rodin independently discovered the original musical frequencies, without knowing it, in his master mathematical Matrix shown in Figure 6.

These specific number wave patterns, Rodin realized, touch every part of reality from black holes to blood cells. All matter, in other words, displays this "signature of God" or math-in-motion at a most fundamental level.

Though you may not perceive material moving at the atomic level, everything is vibrating. The math underlying this movement has been generally disregarded, even suppressed throughout the world for

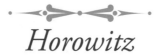

Figure 6. Rodin's Mathematical Matrix

∞   ∞

```
396396396396396396396396396396 3
528528528528528528528528528528 5
741741741741741741741741741741 7
963963963963963963963963963963 9
285285285285285285285285285285 2
417417417417417417417417417417 4
639639639639639639639639639639 6
852852852852852852852852852852 8
174174174174174174174174174174 1
396396396396396396396396396396 3
528528528528528528528528528528 5
741741741741741741741741741741 7
963963963963963963963963963963 9
285285285285285285285285285285 2
417417417417417417417417417417 4
639639639639639639639639639639 6
852852852852852852852852852852 8
174174174174174174174174174174 1
396396396396396396396396396396 3
528528528528528528528528528528 5
741741741741741741741741741741 7
963963963963963963963963963963 9
285285285285285285285285285285 2
417417417417417417417417417417 4
639639639639639639639639639639 6
```

∞   ∞

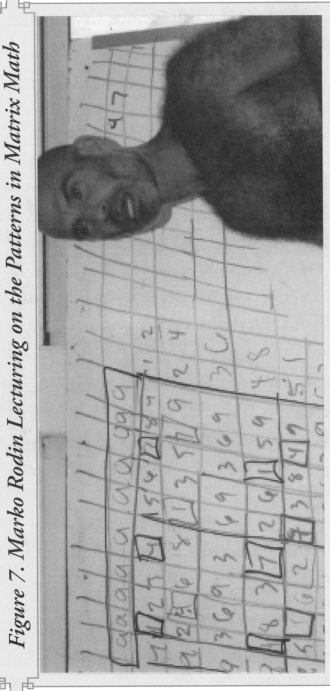

Figure 7. Marko Rodin Lecturing on the Patterns in Matrix Math

The word *pattern* derives from the word "paternal." It means from the seed of the Father. Here, Rodin's math and the patterns he revealed evidences Divine math providing the seed of creation. Mathematicians and physicists who have studied Rodin's work say it provides the basis for revolutionizing energy industries, including the production of free, renewable, non-polluting energy tapping the natural spin-power of the universe. See: www.rodinaerodynamics.org for more details.

millennia. Heralding it now holds the greatest hope for planetary survival. This truth is both spiritually and petrochemically freeing.

In an effort to determine the precise structure of the universe Rodin used the infinity pattern 1,2,4,8,7,5, and a few more sophisticated patterns, to develop the topology of a toroid. According to Rodin's patterns and toroid the numbers 3, 9, and 6—not present in the infinity pattern—actually create the fourth dimension.

Rodin reported the infinity pattern is also produced in the reverse direction offering a bit of insight into the balanced math underlying nature and polarity in the universe.

By simply scanning the Matrix you can observe repeating numbers, 396, 417, 528, 639, 741, 852, 963, 174, and 285—the "Perfect Circle of Sound," the monochord of the universe, with each Hertz frequency deciphering to 9, 3 or 6.

Rodin likens his mathematical map to "God's fingerprint," much like Paracelsus observed during his study of nature. This math appears in the sacred geometry of every facet of the universe. This conclusion is also completely consistent with Plato's and Pythagoras's esteem for the 3, 6, and 9 number set as previously mentioned.

Figure 8. The Infinity Pattern and Separate 3,6,9 Triangle

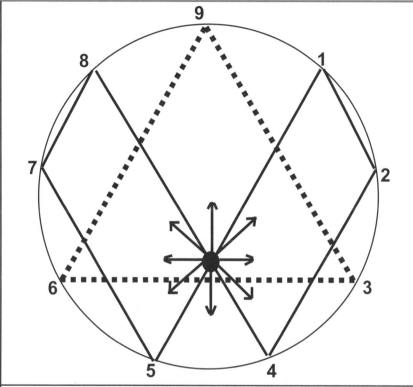

Rodin studied several interesting mathematical patterns. Doubling numbers beginning with 1 yields the pattern 1,2,4,8,7,5 to infinity. Where 1+1=2, 2+2=4 and so on.

The infinity pattern depicted here provides a unidimensional template for multi-dimensional DNA. It also projects the torque and spin of the mathematical Matrix or template of the universe as shown in Figure 9. This simple discovery offers the essential mathematical formula underlying nature, balance, movement, and unity as detailed by Rodin and Haramein.[25]

The numbers 3, 6 and 9 provide a completely distinct triangular pattern which, according to Rodin and others, presents a portal to the fourth dimension, or spiritual realm.

The infinity pattern 1,2,4,8,7,5 diagram is structurally identical to the Standing Gravitational Wave of the universe and, at the microscopic level, your DNA as shown in Figure 10.

LOVE *The Real Da Vinci* CODE

Physicist Nassim Haramein further developed this concept after modifying Einstein's field equations with considerations given to torque, spin, velocity, and polarity. He derived the double toroidal concept of the mathematically perfect universe, as depicted on the next page, to help explain his "Grand Unification Theory."

The implications of these discoveries, like the universe, are limitless and stretch human comprehension. Vastly beneficial creative potential rests in the application of this knowledge to solve civilization's greatest problems. One likelihood, most exciting to both Rodin and Haramein, is the generation of free energy to liberate humanity from petrochemical reliance, economic slavery, and environmental toxicity.

As these toroid structures indicate, the universe is constantly spinning and torquing with energy. Tapping this free-flowing potential was proven possible by Nikola Tesla. His technology was secreted by militarists and energy industrialists. Your mission, should you choose to accept it, is to disseminate this knowledge to help people like Haramein, Rodin, and Müller set humanity free from these deadly demagogues.

After corroborating Rodin's and Haramein's monumental works, many great minds from physics, biology, chemistry, and even computer science, have

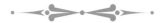

Figure 9. Haramein's Grand Unification Graphic of the Double Toroidal Universe

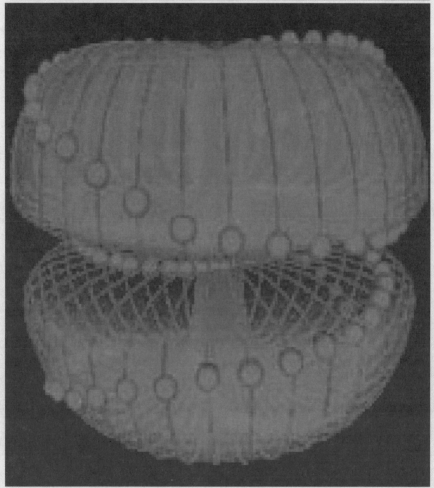

Haramein's thesis reinforces the numerical symbolism discussed earlier—the universe forms mathematically into a spinning figure "8" composed of two polar opposite toroids. This is how and why you attract what you resist and "reap what you sow" in life. This also explains why giving is the same as receiving—"what goes around comes around," or as Forrest Gump said, "Stupid is as stupid does." For Haramein's story, see: http://www.theresonanceproject.org and http://www.theresonanceproject.org/interviews/nassimbayarea.mp3

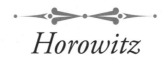

been able to resolve enigmas in their fields by understanding this unique, all encompassing, mathematical system.

In concluding this discussion on the mathematical Matrix, you should realize these core creative energies form the basis for the real Da Vinci Code. This is empirically obvious according to rational deduction from this amassed evidence. This knowledge is inherently empowering and Divinely transformative.

LOVE The Real da Vinci Code opens creativity's communication channel through which sublime inspiration flows. It serves humanity with the enabling mechanism for Divine communion empowering prophetic vision and technological innovation. It is the cosmic Law by which super-humans synchronously live.

Leonardo da Vinci obviously communed with this creative channel. His heart-mind attuned to the relative dimensions of space/time pulling from the future revolutionary ideas and technologies. His world was also largely controlled by religious zealots and dogmatic dictators, but that didn't stop him, nor should it slow you. Leonardo sought how to best benefit humanity through the arts and sciences using this math.

Alternatively, the ignorant masses shall remain clue-

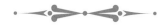

less. Those presented with these profound truths, and who foolishly ignore them, shall miss the blessings available here.

Will you use this information to enable your creative scientific, artistic, and/or technical inventions, or will you allow your motivation to fail for some "good" reason?

By simply applying this knowledge of decrypted mathematics in your life, daily exercising its lawful power; thereby reinforcing this cosmic force of balance within you, you are destined to miraculously fulfill your unique calling.

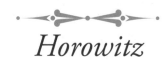
EXERCISES:

1. Get into the habit of thinking like Da Vinci, and living according to the "3s, 6s, 8s, and 9s." Pay reverence to this universal code of creation and the Creator's mathematical musical Matrix by simply counting your actions, or routine operations. Count the number of things that you do. See if you can do them in groups of 3s, 6s, 8s, or 9s.

For example, while brushing your teeth, count the number of times you brush each tooth section, and fix it to this number set. Use 3, 6, 8, 9, or larger harmonics like 12, 15, 17, or 18, that decipher to 3, 6, or 9. Count the number of sips or gulps you take in sequence while drinking. Stop at multiples of 3, 6, 8 or 9. Count the number of steps you take walking to your car. Recalibrate your routine operations so that you end with the miraculous mathematics of creation.

In this way, you will be walking, talking and accessing the Matrix, operating in a manner inherently more creative. This, again, is based on the

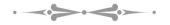
revelation that physical reality manifests (precipitates or crystallizes), in our three dimensional world, from the spiritual domain exclusively accessed through the monochord Matrix of the 3s, 6s, and 9s.

2. Working from right to left, fill in the blanks in the matrix below with the correct numbers.

```
3   63   639   3   63963   6     639   3
52   5   8528   285   852   5    85    85
  4  741   417   174   7   1    41    41
9   39   396   9   39639   3     396    9
28   2   5285   852   528   2    52    52
  1  417   174   741   4   7    17    17
6   96   963   6   96396   9     963    6
85   8   2852   528   285   8    28    28
  7  174   741   417   1   4    74    74
  96   96   963   6   96396   9     963
5   85   8   2852   528   285   8    28
74   7   174   741   417   1   4    74    7
96   963   6   96396   9     963   639
  8  2852   528   285   8    28    28
  174   741   417   1   4    74    74    74
  39   396   9   39639   3    396    96
8   2   5285   852   528   2    52    528
1   417   174   741   4   7    17    17    1
3   63   639   3   63963   6     639   3
52   5   8528   285   852   5    85    85
  4  741   417   174   7   1    41    41
9   39   396   9   39639   3     396    9
28   2   5285   852   528   2    52    52
  1  417   174   741   4   7    17    17
639   39   396   9   39639   3    396
```

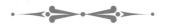

LOVE The Real Da Vinci CODE

Chapter 17
Co-creating Your Reality

Do not fret if it is challenging to comprehend or integrate the full measure of the aforementioned. There is a ton of "food for thought" here. It is natural to need time for digestion and elimination: "out with the old and in with the new." The great news is the mathematical Matrix of creative genius has a subtle way of sneaking up on you. One morning you'll just wake up more musically-mathematically mature and spiritually attuned.

Now it's time to take your next step towards achieving this goal. It's time to explore the concept of creative consciousness that Da Vinci used to the max.

Have you ever wondered how certain life experiences, including synchronistic meetings and miraculous manifestations occur, or how prayed-for outcomes can happen far away in space/time as a result of heart-felt loving intent?

Remember I described DNA as a virtual antennae to Yah? Figure 10 on the next page proves your DNA is vibrationally-entrained to the mathematical Matrix. Even your psycho-neurology is empowered by this supreme energy system. Your thoughts, visions, and imaginings are, likewise, energetically, universally, or cosmically enabled.

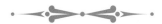

Figure 10. Rodin's Mathematical Infinity Pattern Structurally Identical to Double Helix DNA Segment.

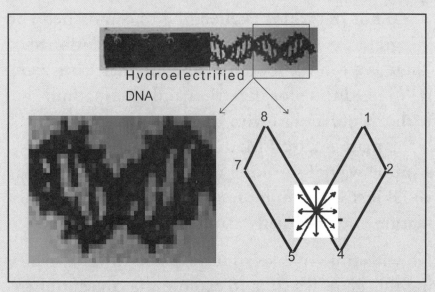

As seen in Figure 8, a diagram of the infinity pattern 1,2,4,8,7,5 is structurally identical to each segment of DNA spiralling in the genetic double helix. Adjacent segments flip sides and polarities to accelerate energy flow and electrogenetic signaling. This animates you with Divine spirit. Again, this same structure appears in Figure 2 in the framework of the Standing Gravitational Wave.

So the mathematics of Divinity is expressed in all creation by Rodin's circular mathematics. This is also evident in The Vitruvian Man as you will soon learn in Chapter 21. "As above, so below." What is true for the macrocosm, is true for the microcosm. The entire universe is perfectly patterned mathematically the same way throughout the *fractal* cosmos. Everything is thusly empowered, enabled, and restored exclusively by Divine mathematical design.[16]

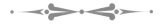
Here is how synchronicities and miracles occur in the lives of people tuned into the Matrix: Frequency transmissions from your heart/mind, as well as your lips, travel throughout the cosmos—the vast spinning figure-8-shaped universe.

As discussed in *Walk on Water*, and you can visualize by examining Haramein's spinning double toroid graphic in Figure 9, once in the Matrix your energized heart-felt messages acquire additional torque, spin, velocity and super-charged polarity. Like magnets they attract their opposite charge, or repel realities similarly charged all based on the Law of this math.

You get whacked when you violate the perfect resonance patterns. That is, you get what you resist and fear, and repel what you fear may be lacking. Our creator does not operate in fear; only by faith, Love and joy.

Dissonance simply attracts itself like a boomerang you throw out into the Matrix. It returns to whack you in the head!

There is nothing to fear, and nothing lacking or broken in the Kingdom of the Heavenly Matrix. So seek this peaceful place of mathematical perfection first. Then you can confidently attract everything you

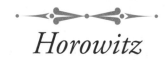

need to survive and thrive. Give every problem with prayer over to the Creator. The Matrix Mastermind knows best how to direct your destiny.

If you desire more money, create wealth as an exercise in applying this real Da Vinci code.

Consider if you resist poverty what happens? You attract more of it due to the negative energy you put out fretting. That negativity feeds the Matrix with dissonance and you get back what you put out. This is much like a computer that runs precisely on mathematically designed crystals. People unfamiliar with operating the system get frustrated with the computer rather than simply taking the time for training. "Garbage in/garbage out!"

Alternatively, you can reap massive wealth. Tithing is a great example. With faith and trust you give and you receive your investment back mathematically multiplied. This is why your tithe is required to make this collaboration and co-creative partnership work.

Again, in addition to supporting my ministry for the work we do on behalf of what is good and just, it blesses you. "Not because I desire a gift: but I desire fruit that may abound to your account." (Philippians 4:17) With your growing support, increasing

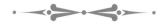

wealth, and tithe, we are additionally empowered to continue this educational effort for earth's physical salvation and people's spiritual evolution.

Everyone will be blessed if you can internalize the justification for collaboration that this knowledge provides. In this way, acting cooperatively and positively versus selfishly and negatively, creatively versus destructively, and collaboratively versus competitively, cuts to the core of creation. Its power spins out to affect the world.

Now you know why the universe is mathematically compelled to respond to your thoughts and imagination, prayers and heart-felt pleas, effecting your creative/attractive or destructive/restrictive outcomes.

This is the technology by which the enlightened you, can either attract or repel life experiences depending on what you transmit, positive or negative.

This best explains karmic law or Divine justice. Spiritual judgment is administered; mathematically compelled by universal balance. Likes repel; opposites attract. Karmically, you get what you need to learn and manifest godliness. If you resist, you get into trouble.

If you are imbalanced, let's say neurotic, you do not need more of the same pathology in your life. So

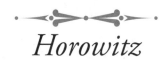
you repel it by seeing the same flaw in others, rejecting them, feuding with them, getting caught up in the energy of your own imbalances; in all cases resistance to Love. This creates this problem's persistence for you and others. The end result is you get to keep, rather than transform like a caterpillar to a butterfly, what you don't like about yourself.

Alternatively, if you are missing something, like an opposite charge, you attract it. . . . Ideal mates and partners attract one another in this way to balance each other's strengths and weaknesses.

This process of rejecting and attracting life experiences, continues until you fill the gaps, or relieve the strain, created by your present lacking as compared with your more complete level of creative abundance through consciousness.

In other words, you are uniquely qualified *and* called to fulfill your spiritual destiny. Transcend dissatisfying deficiency needs now. You have the power, and better things to do in life.

This is the most disheartening aspect of political impositions such as poverty, pestilence, dehydration, and starvation. These are affronts to humanity's capability. The goal is to free yourself so that we free our planet from these scourges to become optimally balanced and loving.

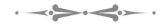

This dynamic also helps explain YahShuah's counsel to seek Heaven first, and how judgment occurs by every word that comes from your mouth. "I tell you this, on the Day of Judgment people will have to give account for every careless word they have spoken; for by your own words you will be acquitted, and by your own words you will be condemned." (Matthew 12:36) Given this book's revelations about language and creative mathematics, this counsel is very wise.

The same seems reasonable for your thoughts and imaginings since these actions are also energetically potent. During these days of spiritual awakening and karmic hastening you can be powerful. But this doesn't guarantee anything but trouble if your actions (which generate vibrations) don't jibe with the math of the Matrix.

Human spirituality and creative consciousness is expanding exponentially due to this massive spiraling sound picking up velocity. Divine attunement and miraculous manifestations is precisely what is ongoing for a growing multitude. Those aware are getting turned on and tuned in to this process of ever-expanding fully-sustaining Love. Those not tuned to the right station just can't hear the music.

Again, if you foolishly ignore this dynamic truth,

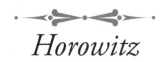

you will not be going with the flow. You will be ignored and will not engage this co-creative opportunity. You simply reap what you sow as part of the problem or solution. *It is nothing or everything when you engage this quest*! It's your choice.

Heed the advice that "the Kingdom of Heaven is near," and you will increasingly experience it. Choose to commune in it, reminding yourself to gratefully receive blessings from Heaven every moment. This is the meaning of Jim Morrison's famous Doors lyric, "Break on thru to the other side."

The math in the real Da Vinci's code is omnipresent and consistent throughout the universe—the macrocosm and the microcosm. Müller found that all celestial bodies and cell organelle, in fact, all of physical creation, share predetermined physical characteristics, intelligent design, based on this underlying code of governing mathematics—the 3s, 6s, 8s and 9s—fundamental to metaphysics. Detailed technical treatments of this important subject are available from Müller and Haramein as directed in the reference section.

Given all of the above, assessing your life status at any moment is simple. You're either flowing with the current in peace and harmony, or treading wa-

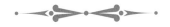
ter exhaustively trying to hold your position against a stronger current. One choice puts you at risk of drowning. The other is optimally freeing. Have you the courage and intelligence to choose wisely?

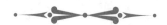

Chapter 18
Recruiting Cells for Co-creating Health

Given the macrocosmic reflection in the micro-cosm it is apparent that Divine intelligence exists at every level of life.

Therefore, it is likely that each cell containing a genetic blueprint of the universe operates with equal metaphysical intelligence. Individually and as groups, your cells may be relied upon, and even recruited, to respond intelligently to disease.

These microscopic allies naturally know how to thrive and provide sustenance. They are naturally attuned to this spiritual input and electromagnetic vibrations. Your cells use math as co-creative stimuli to affect physiologic functions that generate miracu-lous healings.

Positive thinking and visualized prayers turns on the power your cells and tissues need and use for heal-ing.

Miraculous healing is simply a dimension away in Heaven's Matrix. Right now it is recharging your spirit-filled "temple," your body, without you even knowing it. This is the best way to explain why

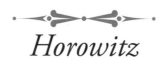

sleep is so refreshing. You are naturally restored by free-flowing energy.

The Matrix also explains why people living in fear, or driven by guilt, get sick. Fear and guilt triggers the "Devil's Tone" disharmonic (interval between the 528Hz and 714Hz frequencies of the mono-chord). These emotions tug at your heart strings and block the flow of Love required for health and longevity. Anger, sadness, and jealousy link your left-brain/ego-mind to this dissonance. Over activity here causes nervous breakdowns. Da Vinci obviously knew this. The Vitruvian Man, you'll notice in Figure 13, is free from appendages in this destructive interval.

The best of life, including your health, depends on your creative imagination, honest communications, and correct lawful orientation to the musical Matrix.

This wholistic paradigm, or mind-body-spirit inter-action with the Matrix, explains psychosomatic reactions.

The Matrix potentiates creative consciousness. This best explains healing by placebo. It also explains placebo's energetic opposite called nocebo.

Most people have heard that a placebo, such as a sugar pill, recommended by someone with perceived authority, prompts healing in more than 30 percent

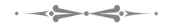

of cases. The deadly opposite is also true for the nocebo. Simply telling a person they are chronically challenged or terminally ill can have devastating affects. As I advanced in *Walk on Water*, nocebo-related ailments are commonly caused by frightfully negative disease labels, poor prognostications, and urgent or deadly professional proclamations. These trigger fear and disease in patients prone to attract what they resist, and grow what they seed with fear.

Yet, people run to their M.D.s, medical deities, for help. Unwittingly, they manipulate their patients to their detriment with disease labels.

For instance, the phrase "terminal illness" kills nearly 30 percent of medical victims. It's better to not get diagnosed than be terminally cursed. I cover this topic effectively in my DVD called IATROGENO-CIDE!

Disease labels actually become illness generators, cofactors, or risk factors, in increasing disease and premature death. Widespread understanding of creative consciousness and free-flowing Matrix energy can help relieve this burden of doctrinal imposition on humanity. Wake up from this deadly deception.

Recognizing the structural mathematics empowering the bio-energetics and sacred geometrics of life, all

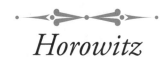

diseases can be addressed simply as *energy blockages* rather than prescribing slash, burn and poison forms of "healthcare."

Soon, people will realize how barbaric modern medicine is. The entire concept of intoxicating the "body electric" with chemical cocktails, and conducting war against biology with risky and expensive antibiotics is recognizably repugnant following recognition of the awesome healing power pouring through the Matrix at every moment.

Obviously, these revelations hold profound potential for transforming the Dark Age of drug-dependence and public confusion. You stand on the threshold of paving the new paradigm with this knowledge.

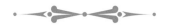

EXERCISES:

1) List at least three unwanted circumstances, repeating patterns, or diseases in your life that you have been attracting or co-creating attitudinally and/or behaviorally.

a)

b)

c)

2) Get into a relaxed and prayerful position. With heartfelt loving intent allow your imagination, or creative consciousness, to commune with the Matrix. This is what master-meditators do when they slow brain wave activity to achieve pure being. In the Judeo-Christian sense, I am talking about allowing the Holy Spirit to flow into you. Allow this vibration for restoration to bathe your cells and body parts with healing energy. Some people see, or experience, this as being bathed with the loving light of God. Others feel this state as a vibration, or hear it as an inner wind or sound of rushing water. The exercise and experience is unique for each person with general similarities.

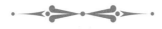

Once you have done this to the best of your ability, prayerfully propose that any remaining disease patterns in your life or body disappear for all time.

3) Joyfully giving thanks, praise, and credit to the Matrix Maker for supporting your prayer(s) and fulfilling your positive intent(ions). Use the space below to write your "thank you note" to the Most High, expressing sincere gratitude and joyful appreciation as though already in receipt of your goal(s):

Chapter 19
Technology for the Communion or Bio-Spiritual Apocalypse

I consider DNA your hardware for Divine communion. There are different types, or species, of DNA just as there are many types of computers. The real Da Vinci code, the mathematical Matrix of the universe is like a widely distributed software program that make all these different computers and DNA species work.

Müller and his collaborators determined that everyone's DNA is in perfect nodal resonance with universal gravity that results from the mathematical-musical Matrix.

Like the pattern seen in figures 8 and 10, DNA's structure is a direct result of the patterned spiraling Matrix of this universe's mathematical design.

In other words, with the universe mathematically unified, lawfully ordered, precisely operating, energetically structured, and musically harmonized with your DNA, tinkering with earth's genetic pool is foolish to say the least. It may be deadly for virtually every living creature.

From Haramein's "Grand Unification Theory," and sacred understanding of the Matrix—the mathematical basis of modern physics and biocosmolo-

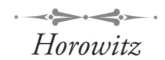
gy—comes recognition of the grossest risk of genetic engineering. The world is now threatened with the apocalypse of pan-generational genome derangements. Devolution of all species seems destined by "unnatural selection." Genetic tinkering threatens food production everywhere. Farmers are losing their organic seed stocks from cross pollinations by bees buzzing from one field to the next carrying man-made mutations.

The way out of this fix is presented here. This decrypted Da Vinci code implores rational genetic conservation for physical salvation, spiritual evolution, and Divine communion.

The evolving New Age or Messianic Age is only possible through widespread revelation that people's hardware and software must be preserved with the Divine program.

In this program, Love is the great healer. To survive and thrive today you must integrate this knowledge of Love central to your mathematical/structural integrity and harmony with the universal unity. Otherwise you will die of spiritual deficiency, also known as a "broken heart." This, along with nutritional fat poisoning, is the leading cause of heart failure.

This is commonly seen with elderly couples where after one spouse dies the other soon follows. There is both a heart-felt spiritual deficiency from the loss of

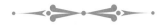

a loved one and physical stress prompting immuno-
logical meltdown.

Man-made mutations oppose natural selection as
dictated by the Matrix and corresponding physics
including the conservation of matter and energy associated with sacred geometry. This universal Law is
being broken daily, in thousands of research labora-
tories and medical clinics around the world. Wher-
ever genetic bioengineering is advancing, prospects
for a free and lawful world are diminishing.

As I documented in *Death in the Air: Globalism,
Terrorism & Toxic Warfare* (June, 2001), the highly
profitable genetics cartel is intimately tied to Big
Pharma and directed by leading energy industrialists. These covert operators plan to control you and
your wages every way possible.

In fact, this profitable bio-ethics violation of the
Matrix's natural selection and vibrational perfection
risks omnicide—global genocide affecting all species.

The Law of the Matrix that empowers nature and
maintains universal integrity by such Divine design
opposes genetic mutations.

Simply consider what happens when you build a
sand castle on a beach at low tide. Sure you can do
it. You can mold this part of nature into the shape
you desire. A little later what happens? The tide

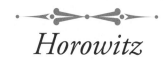

rushes in and washes your castle away. The strength of your castle just can't compete with the ocean's flow.

Likewise, man-made genetic creations are doomed to be short-lived compared to biology controlled by natural selection and evolution. The current exercise of unnatural selection through laboratory creation by Big Pharma produces non-sustainable reliance on typically less hardy species.

In other words, genes were originally vibrated sequentially by nature into their sacred spirals. The same energy that made them is needed to sustain them. Tolerating ignorance and global industrialists' arrogance in the face of dramatic risks is simply insane.

Müller wrote that because DNA's wave form reflects the Standing Gravitational Wave's form, genetic modifications are likely sending distress signals out into the universe. These virtual shock waves transmit throughout the unified field. They move through the double-toroid figure-8-shaped universe where these distress signals pick up torque, spin, and velocity.

This scientific theory is now backed by knowledge of the real Da Vinci code. This code proves intelligent design. It decrees universal unity and integrity of energetic operations based on Matrix music and mathematics. This genetic aspect of the Matrix's

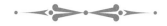

energy and influence demands multi-dimensional or quantum reasoning and holistic responsibility.

This view contrasts sharply with the views of most genetic "experts" serving special interest groups in Big Pharma.

These myopic genetophiles value profits ahead of people and think they can get away with the unnatural injustice of genocide. They are in for a surprise.

There is a rising tide of consciousness rapidly cleansing this planet. Its chief objective is to save valuable resources for posterity.

Vatican researcher Pantaleone said Da Vinci exhorted Pope Leo X to use his inventions only to better humanity. "Leonardo's final message was that although the inventions should be released by the Vatican as necessary, the knowledge of his true identity should be kept a secret until at least 2006, when the world would begin an amazing transformation."

The Spiritual Renaissance Leonardo predicted is unfolding for the fulfillment of humanity's Divine destiny. This outcome is assured like music in the scroll of history. Life is the exclusive property of the monochord Maker. This power and direction shall not be denied.

Can you see more clearly now how and why you obtained this publication? Do you sense a common

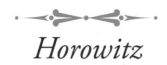

urgency for man and nature? Will you use this knowledge wisely now that we face extinction from non-sustainable consumption and degeneration of everything natural?

Leonardo Da Vinci advanced nearly identical concerns in two drawings completed shortly before his death. Figure 11 reprints the End Times "Cataclysm" brought about by ignorance and official malfeasance.

Figure 12 shows the rarely-viewed little-discussed "Allegory" generating this apocalypse. Here, Da Vinci's Tree of Life is shown uprooted by the global beast—the bull representing the pagan god of power and fertility, Baal. Its craft navigates the oceans of time, abusing the creative elements of wind and water, to direct its booty from organized religion to the heart of the Illuminati. Life is manipulated thusly, through turbulence within the serfdom, to profit the bankers that control land and sea.

Da Vinci personally experienced this Church corruption and conspiracy involving the world's first crime families—the Borgia and the Medici. He witnessed how their great wealth and demonic

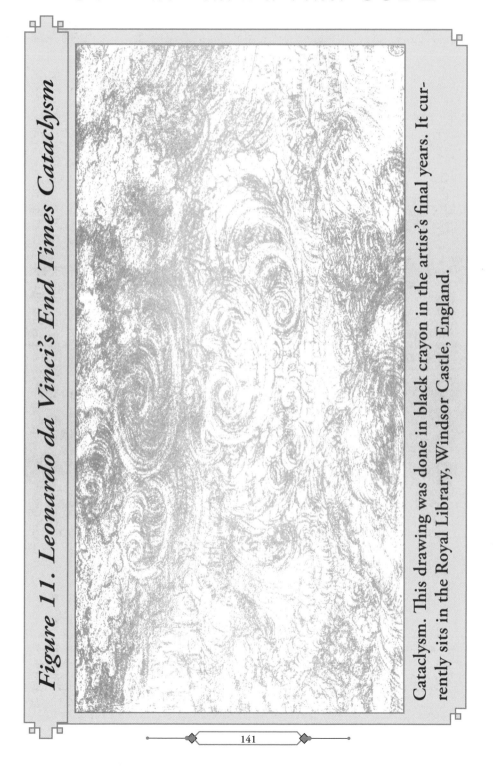

Figure 11. Leonardo da Vinci's End Times Cataclysm

Cataclysm. This drawing was done in black crayon in the artist's final years. It currently sits in the Royal Library, Windsor Castle, England.

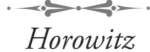

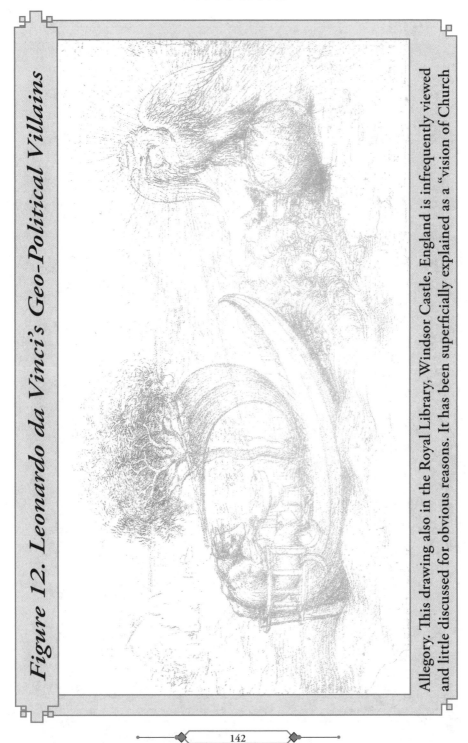

Figure 12. Leonardo da Vinci's Geo-Political Villains

Allegory. This drawing also in the Royal Library, Windsor Castle, England is infrequently viewed and little discussed for obvious reasons. It has been superficially explained as a "vision of Church

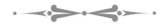

direction influenced the Church, holy wars, and the Royalty's military might. This is symbolized by Da Vinci's eagle comfortably clawing the globe.

Much is written about the nepotism and criminality of the Borgia's Pope Alexander VI who died during his attempt to assassinate a Cardinal. This Pope reigned during Leonardo's most productive years as a military weapons contractor. The Medici crime thereafter took control over Catholic affairs. Pope Leo X, Clement VII, and Leo XI were all members of the Medici family. According to art historians, Figure 12 is "associated with the marriage of Giuliano de' Medici" to Philiberta of Savoy.

From banking, the Medici got into religion, politics, and eventually our heads. This Jewish family played a significant role in history. You may recall from Shakespeare's *Merchant of Venice* that Catholics, including the Popes, were forbidden to lend money for interest, which Jewish bankers did routinely for Christendom.

According to a recent PBS documentary:

> The Medici created a lucrative partnership with . . . the Catholic Church. In what had to be one of the most ingenious enterprises of all time, the Medici bank collected 10% of your earnings for the Church. If you couldn't pay, you faced excommunication - a one-way ticket to hell. The Pope himself had a massive overdraft, and the Medici bank became the most profitable business in Europe. By 1434, half the bank's

revenue came from the 'Rome branch', which was in fact little more than a mobile bank that followed the Pope around the world.

During Da Vinci's time, Medici Leo X was accused of this corruption by Martin Luther which began the reformation at the time of the Medici funded and directed Renaissance.

EXERCISES:

1) Please consider how you might use this knowledge to engage more effectively in life at this most exciting and challenging time—a period of spiritual warfare and renaissance. Meditate on the possibilities of applying this knowledge. Allow yourself to be intuitively and creatively guided.

2) Familiarize yourself with the Holy Harmony CD by going online to: http://www.steam-ventinn.com/holy_harmony. Use the recording containing the "Perfect Circle of Sound" to help you gain your next creative step. Pray for receiving your personal direction in this regard by communing in the Matrix with heartfelt loving and thankful intent. The Source of power to gain your next step to advance important service thrives in this Matrix. Use the space provided on the next two pages to record your insights and creative direction:

Chapter 20
The Law of Entrainment

Consider this question: What compels miracles in a universe ordered mathematically?

The answer is *entrainment*.

Entrainment is defined as "boarding the train." In this case, it is the train carrying the Spiritual Renaissance—the real "Soul Train."

The simplest example of physical entrainment is the eventual synchronizing of menstrual cycles among women living in the same dormitory. This involves synchronizing their physiological, hormonal/neuro-endocrine cycles. Amazing that all of this occurs naturally, directed bio-energetically.

A peaceful world in which people band together aboard the Peace Train, offers great hope and Divine promise. The Matrix commands musical-mathematical entrainment. With this technology humanity is being synchronized in a natural reparative movement. To board the train you simply need to make a commitment of faith, and consistently choose to honor the technology and its Supreme Source. There are zero rational alternatives in a world urgently threatened as ours now is.

Boarding begins now.

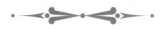
Entrainment expert Joshua Leeds best defines musical "psychoacoustic entrainment." The process reflects your heart-mind's adjustment to the beat of the universe. He describes this as an "important aspect of resonance . . . [that] concerns changing the rate of brain waves, breaths, or heartbeats from" chaotic and stressed to relaxing and harmonious. This is done "through exposure to external, periodic rhythms" or frequencies of sound. This is accomplished by integrating the left brain/right brain balance to augment the heart-mind, and by listening to the sacred tones that resonate throughout the ethers for eternity.

We have entered the miracle millennium Da Vinci predicted. It is no accident the center of the Matrix resonates the third note of the original Solfeggio musical scale. This note is "MI"—as in DO, RE, *MI*—short for "mira gestorum" in Latin, and "miracles" in English. As detailed in DNA: Pirates of the Sacred Spiral (2005), this note is known to miraculously repair damaged DNA. The genetic repair capability of this tone, and the powerful influence it has over everyone, rests assured by the Law of entrainment.

As you will soon learn, 528 Hz relays the color green—the center of the rainbow. This note resonates Love energy throughout the cosmos, and vibrates the center of your heart chakra.

"Universal Entrainment," as I prefer to call it in this context of empowering the Spiritual Renaissance, involves human psycho-emotional and physical resonance—harmonizing with the core creative frequencies or rhythms of the Matrix, akin to tuning into your Divine essence. The Love tone, 528Hz, is vitally important in this regard.

This Divine attunement is precisely what Apostle Paul prescribed in I Corinthians when he wrote the only intimate way to know God is to experience the Spirit of God.

In the exercises at the end of this chapter, I have superimposed on Da Vinci's Vitruvian Man the mathematics of the monochord Matrix and "Perfect Circle of Sound." You can use this knowledge to accelerate your spiritual evolution and Divine entrainment.

The "Perfect Circle of Sound" provides the musical communications for broadcasting Divine communion for the enlightened masses.

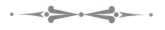
EXERCISES:

1) Using a red pen, place the numbers 1-9 in their appropriate positions adjacent the tones at the outer edge of the circle beginning with "1" above 417Hz. Next, use a ruler to draw: 1) the infinity pattern and 2) a dashed-line representing the 3, 6, 9 Trinity Pattern. Then locate the genetic and physical reproductive center of humans. Next note the position of the umbilicus within your graphic.

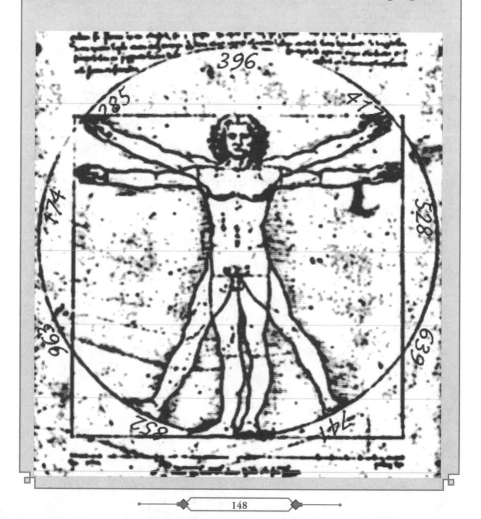

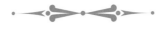
EXERCISES *continued*:

2) Using your pen, and ruler draw a pentagram on the graphic below. Begin with a line across Da Vinci's drawn neck and shoulder line continuing to the two edges of the circle. Connect these two points to the base of each outer foot. Then from here, the star's base, draw two lines to the top of the circle above Vitruvius's head to complete the pentagram.

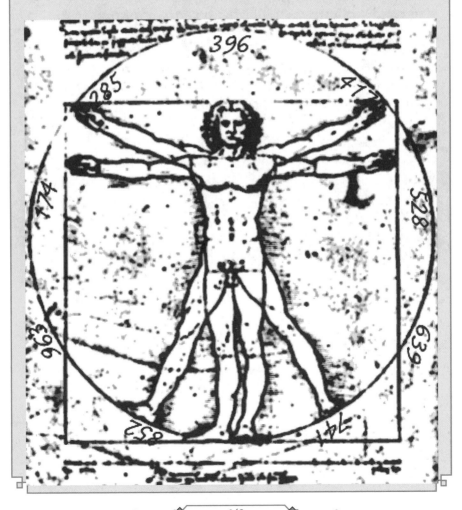

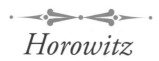

EXERCISES *continued*:

Now turn this book upside down and view the penta-gram you just drew. Examine this symbol for the in-famous Baphomet—the occult symbol for the devil?

According to historians, the Knights Templar were persecuted by the Church for alleged idol worship of the Baphomet featuring the head of the goat. This myth has persisted more than 600 years. Peter Un-derwood's dictionary definition of Baphomet states:

"a deity worshipped by the Knights Templar, and in Black Magic as the source and creator of evil; the Satanic goat of the witches' Sabbath and one of the names adopted by Aleister Crowley."

According to Templar History Magazine, Templars simply see this image as representing "absorption into wisdom." This truth, validated by these real Da Vinci code revelations, was secreted from the time King Phil-ip of France sought to own the vast Templar wealth, and he along with Pope Clement V had the Templars captured and tortured. During these tortures they made false confessions including the disclosure that they had worshipped an idol said to be the Baphomet.

On the next page you can see that the primary sym-bols for the Baphomet, the goat, Freemasonry—in-cluding the compass and ruler—along with Masonry's Grand Union Lodge of England, actually sources from this ancient truth about the mathematical-musical Ma-trix of the monochord and its creative sacred geometry.

Source: http://www.templarhistory.com/baphomet. html

Figure 13. Symbols of Royalty, Freemasonry & Occult

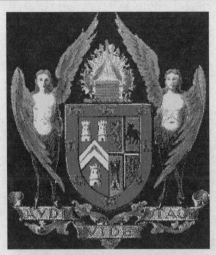

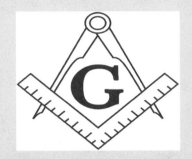

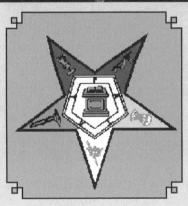

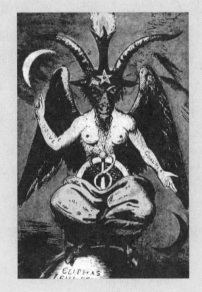

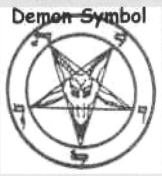

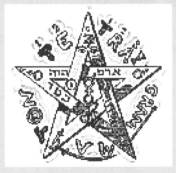

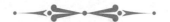

LOVE The Real Da Vinci CODE

Chapter 21
The Vitruvian Man and the Grand Unification

The Vitruvian Man beautifully blends art and science. It was named after the 1st Century B.C. architect and Roman engineer Vitruvius.

Above all of his accomplishments, Vitruvius is known to have heralded water as the source of society and human culture. It is believed that he became Julius Caesar's chief engineer, and following Caesar's death, in 44 B.C., Vitruvius helped direct the construction of the Roman aqueduct water system. His textbook *De Architectura libri decem* (Ten Books on Architecture) survived Classical Antiquity to heavily influence artists and engineers from the Early Renaissance forward.

Like Da Vinci, Vitruvius believed in the supreme importance of mathematics as expressed through architecture, the arts, and sciences. He believed that an architect cannot reach perfection without becoming a pure mathematician and mastering geometry, astronomy, music, and the arts.

The great Renaissance architect Leon Battista Alberti used Vitruvius's ideas in his *De re aedificatoria* (1452, Ten Books on Architecture), and likewise professed as Plato and Phythagoras had previously,

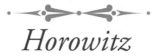
Figure 14. The Vitruvian Man: Communion Matrix Map

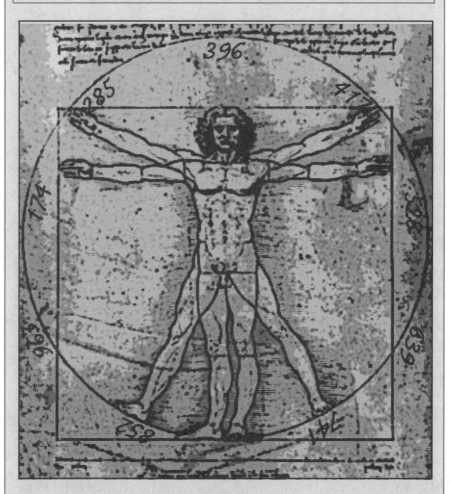

Leonardo da Vinci's famous rendering of the "Universal Man" reaching and stepping "out of the box" to consciously commune with the music of the Matrix. Here the monochord of frequencies in cycles per second is superimposed on the perimeter of the cosmic circle of sound. This "Perfect Circle of Sound" vibrationally establishes physical reality including your human body. At every instant, every atom, molecule, genetic strand, and cell is being reprogrammed, energized, sustained, and entrained beyond your conscious awareness. This revolutionary knowledge brings consciousness to the Divine process of creation.

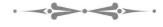

the arts, sciences, and architecture, were all critically governed by mathematical laws and proportions.

Inspired by this knowledge, Leonardo drew The Vitruvian Man. This symbol became *the* icon for natural living and holistic healing. It is a simple drawing depicting The Universal Man with 4 arms, 4 legs, and a head—nine projections altogether extending to the edge of a square representing Earth and a circle representing Heaven and all of creation. The art projects human balance within this perfection. This is what the master genius sought as well as expressed.

Referencing Stanford University's online analysis of this composition:

> This rendering of the Vitruvian Man, completed in 1490, is fundamentally different than others" produced by Da Vinci's architectural and technological mentors. The circle and square image was uniquely overlaid on top of each other to form one image. Without this key adjustment, Da Vinci's predecessors "were forced to make disproportionate appendages.

You will note Da Vinci depicted the cosmic circle representing Heaven and the spiritual domain as a value worth pursuing from the lower earthly vibrational state.

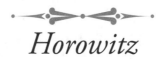

Leonardo's famous drawings of the Vitruvian proportions of a man's body first standing inscribed in a square and then with feet and arms outspread inscribed in a [heavenly] circle provides an excellent early example of the way in which his studies of proportion fuse artistic and scientific objectives.

It is Leonardo, not Vitruvius, who points out that 'If you open the legs so as to reduce the stature by one-fourteenth and open and raise your arms so that your middle fingers touch the line through the top of the head, know that the centre of the extremities of the outspread limbs will be the umbilicus, and the space between the legs will make an equilateral triangle' [with its tip at the groin representing the male creative and procreative element. The female element is positioned at the center of gravity at the umbilicus. The circular spiraling umbilicus is the center point for communing with the cosmos. (Accademia, Venice).

Here Da Vinci provides one of his simplest illustrations of a shifting 'centre of magnitude' without a corresponding change of 'centre of normal gravity'. This remains passing through the central line from the pit of the throat through the umbilicus and pubis between the legs. Leonardo repeatedly distinguishes these *two different 'centres'* of a body, i.e., the centers of 'magnitude' and 'gravity' (Keele 252).

The center of gravity here at the umbilicus metaphorically projects your communion with Creator. Your lifeline of spiritual/energetic sustenance springs from the center of the Matrix to the center of your "holy temple." This concept of rebirthing/recreating

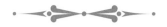
yourself at every moment through Divine communion in the womb of the Matrix with the umbilicus of sound is additionally supported by messages recently found in Hawaiian holy water. This sacred knowledge is detailed more at www.steamventinn.com/breath_of_the_earth.

> "This image provides the perfect example of Leonardo's keen interest in proportion. In addition, this picture represents a cornerstone of Leonardo's attempts to relate man to nature. *Encyclopaedia Britannica* online states, "Leonardo envisaged the great picture chart of the human body he had produced through his anatomical drawings and Vitruvian Man as a cosmografia del minor mondo (cosmography of the microcosm). He believed the workings of the human body to be an analogy for the workings of the universe." (Source: http://leonardodavinci.stanford.edu/submissions/clabaugh/history/leonardo)

I added emphasis in the previous quote to draw your attention to the 3, 6, and 9 triangle formed in The Vitruvian Man. As he stands, the pinnacle of the triangle is at his groin as the "center of magnitude." The "center of gravity" is above this representing the higher female values. Indeed, as Da Vinci well understood, this polarity of male/female biocosmography sources from the monochord/Matrix transmitting the "Perfect Circle of Sound."

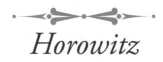
This analysis of The Vitruvian Man, even by mainstream media, scientists, architects, and historians, validates this comprehensive decryption of this most esoteric Da Vinci work. The drawing is a cryptographic higher-self portrait memorializing Da Vinci and his recognition of a Universal Spirit and Divine Source.

The above analysis of the Vitruvian Man also supports my thesis that Da Vinci's code for mastering the mathematics of language and life heralds your capacity to commune with the Creator through the Matrix. The Vitruvian Man encrypts the fundamental mathematics and tonal dynamics required for the "Grand Unification." Da Vinci himself demonstrated this.

Given this knowledge, you can supercharge your link to Divine Source by realizing, that is *making real*, your true identity in the Grand Duality, as both creator and created. You are this mystical miracle. You came from this music and return to it. Get it? *You are this music*!

Your essence in Matrix music calls forth your spirit to live in harmony with the universal symphony, to drop your false notion(s) of separation, to *embrace unification*.

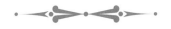

LOVE *The Real Da Vinci* CODE

The best artists, especially musicians and vocalists, flow with their music. . . . In the moment of performance they become their creations and compositions. They commune or entrain with their creations in the spirit of Love.

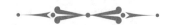

LOVE The Real Da Vinci CODE

Chapter 22
The Real Da Vinci Code
and the "Perfect Circle of Sound"

As shown in Figure 16, there is a spiraling pentagonal geometry linked to the "Perfect Circle of Sound." This lays out upon the Vitruvian Man so well it can not be an accident. His heart is centered adjacent the 528 Hz frequency of Love. His umbilicus is centered within the pentagons. Also, his feet that are stepping out of the box appear to indicate a clockwise spin, or continuous rotation, much like the ascending pentagon-producing musical scale shown in this figure. This is also true for double helix DNA viewed from its center. All of this evidences the "cosmografia del minor mondo" that Da Vinci researched and expressed.

Music is the source of the 5-pointed sacred geometry in Figure 16 and Da Vinci' famous drawing. The pentagram has been classically associated mathematically with the phi ratio (See: www.intent.com/sg1). The sacred secret within Da Vinci's Vitruvian Man is reconciled with knowledge of the "Perfect Circle of Sound." The master monochord of the Creator's Matrix is laid out here as Leonardo's cosmographic encryption.

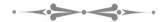

Figure 15. The Vitruvian Man as a Cryptograph of the Human–Cosmic Monochord

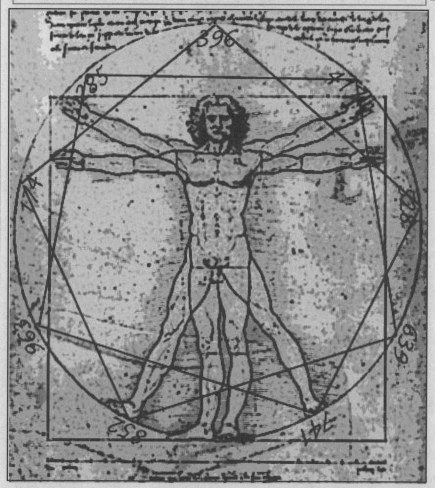

The circular monochord heralded by Pythagoras, Plato, Vitruvius, Da Vinci and others engaged in mystery-school education is decrypted here in service to humanity's psychosocial and spiritual evolution toward the Grand Unification. The goal of mystery scholars was optimal heavenly communion using this monochord. Their knowledge was based on fundamental musical-mathematics featuring the "Perfect Circle of Sound" that vibrates life and physical reality into crystalline existence. This creative impetus operates as a virtual umbilical chord spiraling electromechanically between your body and the mathematical Matrix of the universe. This Divine creative technology, this musical-mathematics, is fundamental to profound advances occurring in physics and the physical sciences. This image is a metaphor for the macrocosmic/microscopic order of the fractal universe.

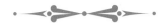

Figure 16. Cross Section of Double Helix DNA: Sacred Geometry of Pentagrams

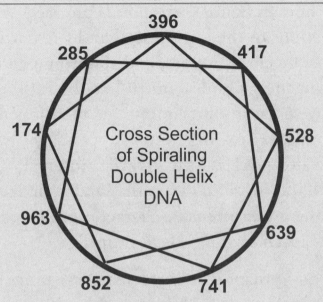

396

285   417

174   528

Cross Section
of Spiraling
Double Helix
DNA

963

639

852   741

The figure above results from connecting keys in the "Perfect Circle of Sound" that correspond to the ascending or descending tones matching Rodin's mathematical infinity pattern as shown in Figure 8. This is also consistent with Phi (or Golden Mean) ratio analysis. The lower figures show the sacred geometry of pentagrams that reflect the macrocosmic/microscopic order of the fractal universe.

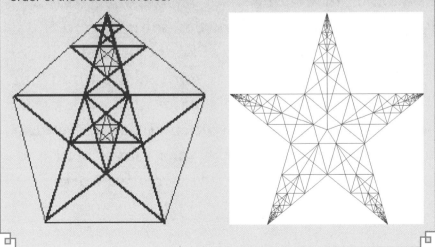

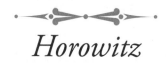

You will notice each of many reference lines in Da Vinci's human figure corresponds precisely with intersections of the key musical and geometric elements—the circle, square, and spinning pentagon. These are energy nodes, much like the In(6) in which we creatures precipitate. As mentioned, Da Vinci omitted drawing human appendages between 528 Hz and 741Hz—the "Devil's interval." This was a choice made to direct the Divine in people versus the lower offensive character produced when humans reach for the "Devil's tone."

Plato and Pythagoras considered these tones and the phi ratio as sacred. Each larger or smaller section correlates with the phi ratio raised or lowered by the whole note/number scale. That is, phi, phi2, phi3, etc.

As detailed in *Healing Codes for the Biological Apocalypse,* the original ancient Solfeggio musical scale—the "Perfect Circle of Sound"— holds major implications for humanity's spiritual evolution and civilized ascension. For this reason this work has been moving musicians, mathematicians, physicists, and other researchers worldwide to investigate and integrate these findings in their creative works.

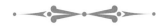

LOVE The Real Da Vinci CODE

The "Perfect Circle of Sound" has been increasingly associated with profound outcomes, miracles included! Read the testimonials posted on http://www.steamventinn.com/holy_harmony. These describe people's experiences from listening to these special tones. What might you expect from listening to the Creator's music?

Recall I mentioned the third note—MI—transmits Love, the 528Hz frequency. It is characterized by, or capable of, producing miracles, according to its definition in *Webster's Dictionary*:

MI–ra gestorum (Miracle)–pronounced "me"

1. *an extraordinary occurrence that surpasses all known human powers or natural forces and is ascribed to a divine or supernatural cause esp. to God.* 2. a superb or surpassing example of something; wonder, marvel [1125-75]; ME <L Miraculum=Mira(Ri) to wonder at. *fr* (French): sighting, aiming to hold against the light. (gestorum: gesture; movements to express thought, emotion; any action, *communication*, etc. intended for effect.)

This note warms people's hearts. You've heard the phrase, "Home is where the heart is." This tone summons us home through the universal umbilical chord of sound to commune with our grand Creator and naturally with each other. MI transmits near the center of the "Perfect Circle of Sound," and near the center of the mathematical Matrix of the universe.

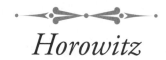

Zero chance an accident, Da Vinci's Vitruvian Man, superimposed onto the "Perfect Circle of Sound," places this note nearest this icon's heart.

The power and glory of miracle-making with Love and joy is resonating from the center of the universe through your heart. That's why exercising and developing your heart-mind is so important.

These revelations help to explain Da Vinci's deep Love for humanity as well as his Divine creativity. They prove life's core sustaining vibration is Love according to advancing mathematics, physics, and anthropological metaphysics.

The original Solfeggio musical scale, used by Babylonian and Levite priests alike to produce miracles, apparently including three complementary keys, (i.e., 963, 174, and 285Hz) completes the "Perfect Circle of Sound." This music supplies you with more than your holy creative loving spirit. This melodious Matrix music relays the full meaning and blessing of the Vitruvian Man. It offers direction for personal development, spiritual ascension, and optimal communion with the Source of everything.

In *Walk on Water*, I credited toning expert, Jonathan Goldman, for intuiting, "the use of these tones . . . creates a sacred spiral that seems to encode itself as a matrix upon the cellular structure, and particu-

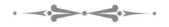

larly on the DNA. I believe this is the Matrix of the 'higher' human—helping create an evolutionary step in our genetic encoding." When Goldman wrote this, he was unaware of the mathematical Matrix described herein.

Goldman further reported that playing these tones in ascending or descending order, "seems to have the ability to nullify any frequencies that are counter productive to our highest good. These frequencies create a blanket of Divine sounds that may counter the effects of harmful energy including bacteria and viruses." The same might be said for all pathology, since, as YahShuah said, "There is nothing missing or broken in the Kingdom of Heaven."

These tones characterize the wholeness and holiness of the Kingdom of Heaven. They amplify your essential resonance, and entrain your physical presence to the Divine. These are the sounds of silence that broadcast eternally. These keys are inherently balancing and universally sustaining. They unlock floodgates for unprecedented restoration and healing.

It is written in Psalm 91:1, "He that dwelleth in the secret place of the Most High shall abide under the shadow of the Almighty." This secret place is the Matrix in which you are well advised to dwell.

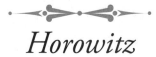

"Without making medical claims," Goldman wrote, "these frequencies likely nullify and dissipate disharmonious energies that may be trying to establish themselves upon our physical, mental, emotional, or spiritual essences. . . . . People call this stress and disease," as these defiant energies ultimately result in injuries and maladies.

"Behold, I give unto you power to tread on serpents and scorpions, and over all the power of the enemy: and nothing shall by any means hurt you." (Luke 10:19)

Goldman's assertions have been substantially supported by research. For example, the frozen water micro-crystal hexagon shown in Figure 17 was photographed by world renowned water researcher and award-winning humanitarian, Dr. Masaru Emoto. The water resonated into this sacred structure during 24-hours of exposure to the "Perfect Circle of Sound" toned and chanted under Goldman's direction on the Holy Harmony CD. (See www.healthyworlddistributing.com.)

Listen to Holy Harmony and experience its affects for yourself, including the restructuring of your body water. This can have a profoundly positive influence on your state of mind, emotions, imaginative capacity, intuitive capability, health, healing, and ge-

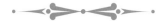

Figure 17. Water Cluster Formed During Exposure to the "Perfect Circle of Sound" on the Holy Harmony CD

This crystal water cluster was photographed in Dr. Masaru Emoto's Japanese laboratory. This structure developed sonically from cube-structured distilled water. The physical transformation occurred during 24 hours of exposure to the vibrations of the "Perfect Circle of Sound."

Toning artist and sound healing expert, Jonathan Goldman,

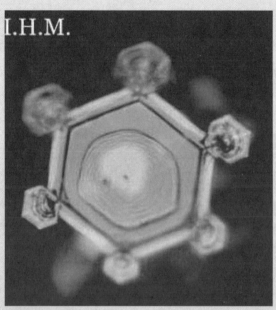

recorded the tones of the real Da Vinci code on a CD entitled Holy Harmony. He used the nine notes in ascending and descending order, directing professional vocalists using tuning forks. The sacred chant he used was the Hebrew letters of the Messiah's name. These photographs show the central portion of this cluster is marked by sound rings made as the water froze.

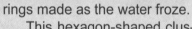

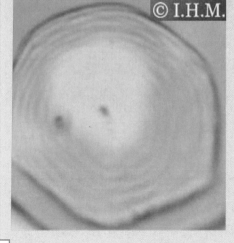

This hexagon-shaped cluster is typical of harmonically energized structured water. Goldman, and numerous other musicians and vocalists worldwide are currently composing additional music for personal and planetary healing based on this knowledge of The Real Da Vinci Code..

Source: http://www.steamventinn.com/holy_harmony.

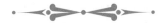

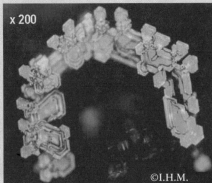

x 200

©I.H.M.

This series of structured water photographs was also taken under the direction of Dr. Masaru Emoto. They show the effects on water structure from a 24-hour exposure to 3E™ sticker resonance. Dr. Emoto reported these structures as "very interesting," as the first shows a well defined arch, typical of matter evolving from the

Fibonacci Series, Phi ratio and Golden Mean math. Notice the sub-structures that resemble the Infinity Pattern in Rodin's math and genetic substructuring.

The crystal on the right side is photographed with a highly unusual halo around it suggestive of an aura or associated energy field. ....

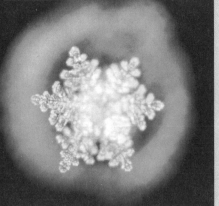

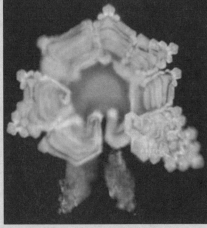

The third crystal cluster appears as a cartoon-like character with hands posed in what looks like prayer. Dr. Emoto's legitimate thesis—that water relays messages, and responds to consciousness, including prayer and loving heart-felt intent—has been criticized by ignorant scientists and blindly-biased reporters. According to revelations in *LOVE The Real Da Vinci CODE*, given water's elemental mathematics, and sacred tetrahedron geometrics, this substance must be respectfully recognized as holding and relaying consciousness as the premier creative medium. Source: http://www.3epower.us.

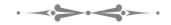
netic expression. The reason for this genetic affect is this kind of structured or "clustered" water has been scientifically determined to be responsible for most of your DNA's electrogenetic influence. (See: *DNA: Pirates of the Sacred Spiral* for more details.)

More evidence is shown in the crystal structures shown in Figure 18, also photographed in Dr. Emoto's lab. This sacred geometry was produced from cube-structured distilled water energetically affected by the "Perfect Circle of Sound" imprinted on the 3E™—Evolutionary Energy Enhancer—sticker. (See: www.3epower.us)

These photographs in figures 17 and 18 help demonstrate the great potential we hold to impact the waters of the world, and all of life, with technologies developed from these simple understandings. (See: http://www.liveh2o.org for more information.)

Given that your body is mostly water, these sacred sounds can vibrate your body water, DNA, and whole person back into harmony with your purest-spiritual self. Imagine the potential for resuscitating and sustaining planet-wide positivity based on these revelations.

Dr. Emoto concludes water receives and transmits mathematical messages. In fact, the material itself makes an obvious statement about human conscious-

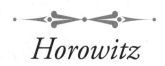
ness. As a creative liquid, here before Earth's creation (Genesis 1:2), the statement water makes about life on Earth, and creative consciousness, is expressed in its three states: solid, liquid, and gas:

Rock solid ice is like hard-headed people. They are fearfully fixed in divisive beliefs, attitudes, and positions. They don't move very much, nor get very far in life, generally speaking. Socially "cold," they are considered less conscious or entirely unconscious.

Heat the ice up a bit and it liquefies and spreads. Flowing water avoids obstacles, and moves along paths of least resistance. It takes direction from nature to commune with its neighbors in the rivers and oceans of life. Conscious spiritually-evolving people do similarly in their inspired lives.

Add more heat, or use the 3E™ and the "Perfect Circle of Sound" to increase the vibrations of water, and your creative medium becomes more etherial or spiritual just like boiling water turns to steam.

Consciousness today, like steam, is rising and spreading. The rainwater that forms from evaporation cleanses and renews the planet. Likewise, as human awareness grows Earth shall be cleansed and renewed. All natural processes and substances, in-

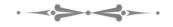
cluding water and creative consciousness best serve to uplift the human spirit to commune, refresh, and renew in the musical-mathematics of pure Oneness.

Figure 19. Messages in the "Breath of the Earth"— Umbilical Chord to the Matrix for Loving Creation

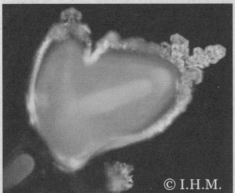

© I.H.M.

The Big Island of Hawaii is famous for its active volcano and powerful purgative and creative energy. Local holy-persons, Kahunas, say the top of Mauna Kea bears the umbilical chord to the entire universe. This is akin to The Vitruvian Man's navel connecting to the center of the cosmos.

These unique structures are part of a larger series of crystals photographed in Dr. Emoto's lab analyzing the "Breath of the Earth™"—lava-heated steam from the Steam Vent Health Retreat. These crystals tell the same loving story about creation. A heart-shaped crystal holds two swords forming a "V" for the Divine feminine principle. The swords mimic those in the Knights Templar medallion shown in Figure 5.

The crystal on the right shows a 12-pointed star with an extraordinary center. Moving from the darkness into the radiant light is a spiriling string of hexagons (the basic structure of organic chemistry and molecular biology). It appears as an umbilical cord might, connecting Heaven

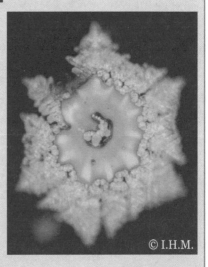

© I.H.M.

to Earth; from the dark formless abyss into the light center of life.

This cluster shows a fetus-like structure with an umbilical cord attached to its navel. Given this accumulating evidence, Dr. Emoto's scientific critics should silence their objections. See http://www.steam-ventinn.com/breath_of_the_earth and www.masaru-emoto.net

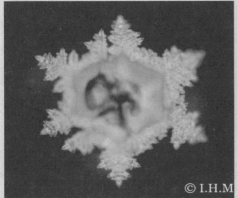

© I.H.M

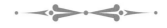
EXERCISES:

List at least three goals or projects in your life that might be aided by employing this new creative knowledge of the "Perfect Circle of Sound."

1)

2)

3)

Write a brief explanation of how the "Perfect Circle of Sound" might help you achieve your goals, or complete your personal project(s), to achieve greater success.

EXERCISES:

Consider the number of people in your life that might appreciate having this knowledge as a creative blessing for personal empowerment, professional success, and enhanced social service. List these people below and set a date by which you will contact them with this information:

Chapter 23
Making This Technology Work For You

Please recall from your Bible study, that the world began when the Creator's "word" acted on water. That is, sound frequencies based on the musical-mathematics were applied to water.

If you were created in the image of God, then your lips must also be creative instruments. For you to evolve yourself and this world with Love and Divine energy, you must, therefore, speak, sing, chant, play or otherwise apply these core creative musical tones to your creative endeavors.

Knowledge of the real Da Vinci code can significantly impact your life. This knowledge proves your personal stresses, psycho-emotional strains, and physical illnesses source from violating the musical-mathematics of the Matrix. Only crazy people go against this fundamental Law.

Simply summarized, all diseases and discords stem from going out of tune with these core creative tones. You may simply require a tune-up to remain optimally healthy, happy, wealthy, and productive. After all, the real Da Vinci code offers unlimited creativity and musical-mathematical access to the Creator's domain—the heavenly Matrix.

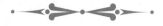

LOVE *The Real Da Vinci* CODE

As you come to rely on this knowledge and its Source for your sustenance, you will become increasingly creative and resourceful.

The real Da Vinci code is fundamental to creationistic science, healing, economic success, spiritual evolution, and planetary salvation. Its unique sounds fill the Kingdom of Heaven, and you, with Love. Entraining with this Matrix brings you heart-to-heart, in intimate contact, with the Spirit of God.

To make this technology, this Divine code, work for you, simply play with the numbers, sacred symbols, sounds, and music described herein. Test the various products and technologies advancing with this wisdom. Increasingly integrate these sacred sounds that entrain humanity Divinely through this mathematical-musical Matrix. You will either perceive this fruit as sweet and nurturing or not. In the stillness of your mind, and the opening of your heart, this harvest of creative genius is increasingly available.

Chapter 24
Summary and Invitation for Collaboration

The root word of education is *educare*, meaning to "lead out [of ignorance] from within." This refers to the special skills and talents each of us acquires by spiritual blessing at birth through the Divine Matrix.

How sad that today's educational institutions are so inept in celebrating this core virtue. Their indoctrination of students with information that is wholistically retarding rather than spiritually freeing is stifling and intolerable. Will you help change it? If so, what might you use and recommend to replace education with educare?

The scientific evidence advanced herein proves the truest Source of your personal freedom comes spiritually from within.

You are a Divine offspring. By nurturing your seedlings, feeding them organically, and loving them optimally they naturally grow inspired by Heaven's ambient music recharging Earth at every moment. Working together in this way we can free humanity's latent talents to develop leadership and creativity for social sustainability.

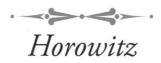

I pray this will be our collaborative quest for the coming years. That you will join our growing team, and contribute to humanity's *edutainment*. Contact www.DrLenHorowitz.com for updates, scheduled events, and to make arrangements for lectures in your area.

Now that you are aware of this most valuable creative technology, you might consider yourself on par with Bill Gates. This knowledge can create opportunity like Gates actualized in his garage. Microsoft's master realized his exclusive knowledge could revolutionize computing and global communications. After integrating the information in this book, you might realize this knowledge, and technologies spun from it, can revolutionize every field of research and development.

Using this knowledge you too can invent new products, innovative methods, revolutionary materials, and Divinely-inspired services.

Essentially, these revelations are part of a popular revolution hastening Spiritual Renaissance.

You can help this revolution by applying this knowledge in practical ways. By developing, and/or distributing, marketing, and selling this knowledge, related products, educational seminars and confer-

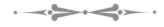

ences, you can make a big positive difference promoting this metamorphosis.

The 3E™ is a simple illustration of how this extraordinary knowledge can be applied to pioneering technologies for better health and living. (See: http://www.3epower.us) Let your imagination flow while inventing additional beneficial products based on this knowledge. You will help everyone by doing so.

As mentioned, musicians worldwide are contributing new music, musical products and instruments. Entrepreneurs are productively engaging this revolution now with related technologies based on the real Da Vinci code

This book is a gift to the world. The financial opportunity here is huge. You can prosper with these well-kept secrets especially by giving and receiving from this treasure for humanity's benefit.

The truth about the Vitruvian Man cryptograph is very beneficial and enabling. Many people perceive an *urgent* need for healing technologies and knowledge to protect and sustain life. With our very existence endangered, the real Da Vinci code appears to be critical for this miracle.

This book is a call to you for action. More research

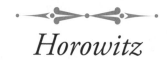

obviously needs to be done and many new products developed. The humanitarian scope of this project includes wealth-building. How else can we get the job done? Everything right comes with sustainability and prosperity.

The Bible foretells that in the "End Times" the "meek shall inherit the Earth and all its riches." The word meek implies loving and gentle. With the Creator's technology, loving spirit-filled people will gain victorious advantage to win in the end.

This previously secreted knowledge levels the playing field in creative mastery. Together, we can take control of this planet, attract massive wealth, restore public health, and co-create sustainable industries for an eco-friendly planet. We had the Industrial Age and the Computer Revolution. Now, be part of the "Matrix Generation."

If you have already received benefits from this instruction, then share it with others. You already listed their names in a previous exercise. Your sharings will expand everyone's blessings, including your own.

Help make people aware of this book and spiritual revolution; fill our "edutaining" events with kindred spirits and conscious persons; become a distributor of *LOVE The Real Da Vinci CODE* and other

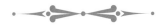

LOVE The Real Da Vinci CODE

Healthy World Distributing, LLC products. Get on our e-mail list by going to: www.lovetherealdavinci-code.com.

This is *not* an invitation to join another network-marketing organization. This is an opportunity to fulfill a very special destiny to make a huge difference in the world and earn substantial income for yourself through a standard limited partnership agreement.

For more information about setting up your association account today, or help with online administration, call 1-888-508-4787, or email tetra@tetrahedron.org.

More Opportunites for Collaboration

Consider your unique talents and interests. Conceive of ways to express yourself creatively in this collaborative venture. Inventions based on these revelations are required in all fields including education, communications, healthcare, physics, agriculture, architecture, fashion, construction, music and more.

When I first conceived of the 3E™ as a novel way of energizing water and people's bodies with the "Perfect Circle of Sound," I then realized the opportunity to literally baptize the entire planet to advance creative consciousness and Divine communion. From

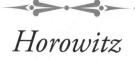

this idea came efforts to send these precise sound signals into the atmosphere and oceans as friends and colleagues are now doing around the world. Can you think of a better way of directing and empowering our prayers for uplifting our planet?

If this sounds strange to you, as it might to newcomers to this great news, reflect on what John the Baptist accomplished with his unique hydrotherapy. Applying this code may be crucial to freeing humanity from Dark Ages mentality. This information is educationally imperative to the whole human family.

3E™s, Holy Harmony CDs, the "Perfect Circle of Sound" tuning fork set, the monochord wind chimes, and the Breath-of-the-Earth™ energized Hawaiian holy water are all products you can use as creative examples. All of these products use the same mathematics and harmonics to impart the core creative frequencies for better health and living.

Powerful messages of Love, thanks, peace, health, prosperity and more may be programmed into your life. Virtually anything and everything in physical reality may be blessed using these Divine revelations in musical mathematics. Bring me your ideas; and I will do my best in collaboration to bring them successfully to market.

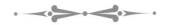

LOVE The Real Da Vinci CODE

Near the beginning of this book I promised to provide technology, even supernatural ways and means, to live your life prosperously and creatively empowered. *LOVE The Real Da Vinci CODE* has achieved this goal. The next step is yours.

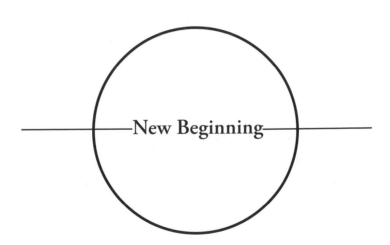

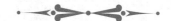

LOVE The Real Da Vinci CODE

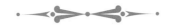

About the Author

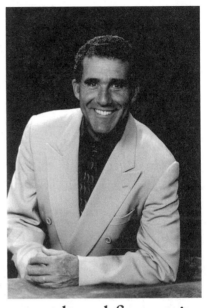

D r. Leonard G. Horowitz (Hebrew name, Arya ben Schlomo ha Levi) is an internationally known authority in public health, behavioral science and emerging diseases.

In 1999, he was voted Author of the Year by the World Natural Health Organization for his monumental research and first national bestseller, *Emerging Viruses: AIDS & Ebola—Nature, Accident or Intentional?*

In 2006, he was honored by the World Organization for Natural Medicine as a "World Leading Intellectual."

In November, 2006, synchronous with the e-book release of *LOVE The Real Da Vinci CODE*, his 16th book, he was honored for his global efforts to advance public health through natural medicine by officials of The Sovereign Orthodox Order of the Knights Hospitaller of Saint John of Jerusalem. This organization was formed in the eleventh century and still operates today internationally for the purpose of healing the sick and protecting the public from emerging health risks.

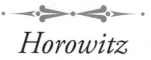

Horowitz

Dr. Horowitz received his doctorate from Tufts University School of Dental Medicine in 1977. As a student at Tufts, he taught medical and dental histology, graduated with honors, and was then awarded a research fellowship in behavioral science at the University of Rochester.

He later earned a Master of Public Health degree from Harvard University focused on behavioral science and media persuasion technologies, and a Master of Arts degree in health education/counseling psychology from Beacon College/Interface Foundation. He served on the research faculty at Harvard School of Dental Medicine to study psychosocial factors in oral health and disease prevention.

While in Boston, he also taught master's candidates, "Pain, Fear and Stress Management" for Leslie College's Institute for the Arts and Human Development.

For more than a quarter century Dr. Horowitz has directed a non-profit educational publishing company that evolved into Tetrahedron, LLC .

Dr. Horowitz's published works include:

• *Emerging Viruses: AIDS & Ebola—Nature, Accident or Intentional?* , the American best-seller now considered a medical classic;

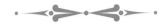

LOVE The Real Da Vinci CODE

• *Healing Codes for the Biological Apocalypse* which permanently expanded the field of therapeutic musicology;

• *Healing Celebrations: Miraculous Recoveries Through Ancient Scripture, Natural Medicine and Modern Science* (2000), which provides practical information and advice for preventing illnesses and protecting individuals through natural-healing;

• *Death in the Air: Globalism, Terrorism and Toxic Warfare,* released three months before the attacks of 9/11, this prophetically-titled critically-acclaimed book examines leading global industrialists' successful efforts to direct contemporary culture through propaganda wars, toxicity, petrochemical/pharmaceutical malfeasance and economic dependence.

• *DNA: Pirates of the Sacred Spiral,* his 2004 book reviewed the science of electrogenetics that speaks to humanity's fundamental spirituality.

Likewise, his 2006 release, *Walk on Water,* advances the mathematics, music, and physical mechanics of the ongoing Spiritual Renaissance. Revelations in this book were foundational for *LOVE The Real Da Vinci CODE,* particularly the pioneering thesis on hydrocreationism that Dr. Horowitz advances.

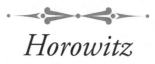

Horowitz

Aside from helping to organize LiveH2O, an international Concert for the Living Waters, and his speaking schedule, Dr. Horowitz oversees the Steam Vent Inn & Health Retreat on the Big Island of Hawaii, where one of the world's most powerful natural healing resources—volcanically-heated steam—is being used to demonstrate Divinity to humanity.

For more information about Dr. Horowitz visit his official website at http://www.drlenhorowitz.com.

Other Dr. Horowitz affiliated sites include:
http://www.healthyworlddistributing.com;
http://www.3epower.us;
http://www.originofAIDS.com;
http://www.C-CURE.net;
http://www.healingcelebrations.com;
http://www.tetrahedron.org;
http://www.liveh2o.org;
http://www.steamventinn.com;
http://www.steamventinn.com/holy_harmony;
http://www.steamventinn.com/breath_of_the_earth;
http://www.bbsradio.com; and
http://www.lovetherealdavincicode.com

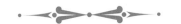

LOVE The Real Da Vinci CODE

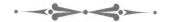

LOVE The Real Da Vinci CODE

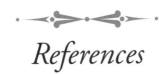

References

Anderson, Warren D. 1994. Music and Musicians in Ancient Greece. Ithaca: Cornell University Press.

Bailhache P. "Music translated into Mathematics: Leonhard Euler", translation from French by Joe Monzo; and "La Musique, une pratique cachée de l'arithmétique?", an article on the musical writings of Leibniz; both available at http://bailhache.humana.univ-nantes.fr/thmusique.html.

Barbera, A. "The Consonant Eleventh and the Expansion of the Musical Tetractys: A Study of Ancient Pythagoreanism", Journal of Music Theory, V. 28, n2, 1984.

Benson, D. Mathematics and Music, http://www.math.uga.edu/~djb/math-music.html (text can be viewed and downloaded in its entirety), 2002.

Bernal, Martin. 1987. Black Athena: the Afroasiatic Roots of Classical Civilization. Vol. I of The Fabrication of Ancient Greece 1785-1985. London: Free Association Books.

Bulckens, Anne M. 1999. The Parthenon's Main Design Proportion and its Meanings. Ph.D Thesis, Geelong, Victoria, Deakin University.

Campbell, Joseph. 1990. The Flight of the Wild Gander: Explorations in the mythological dimension. New York: Harper Perennial.

Chappell, William 1874. The History of Music. (Art and Science.) Vol. I: From the earliest records to the fall of the Roman empire... London: Chappell & Co.

Chatwin, Bruce. 1987. The Songlines. London: Jonathan Cape.

Chén Cheng Yih, ed. 1994. Two-tone Set-Bells of Marquis Yi. Singapore: World Scientific.

Comotti, Giovanni. 1989. Music in Greek and Roman Culture. Trans. Rosario V. Munson. Baltimore and London: Johns Hopkins University Press.

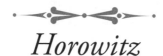

Cornford, Francis M. 1952. Principium sapientiae: The origins of Greek philosophical thought. Cambridge: Cambridge University Press.

Doczi, György. 1981. The Power of Limits: Proportional Harmonies in Nature, Art, and Architecture. Boston and London: Shambhala.

Eliade, Mircea. 1964. Shamanism: Archaic Techniques of Ecstasy. Trans.Willard R. Trask. London: Routledge & Kegan Paul.

Elkin, Adolphus P. 1946. Aboriginal Men of High Degree. Sydney: Australasian Publishing Co.

Farley, Bruce. Blessing the world's waterways: Climate crisis. *Mandala*, a Tibetan Buddhist Journal. October/November 2006; 15-19.

Franklin, John Curtis. 2002a. Terpander: The Invention of Music in the Orientalising Period. Ph.D dissertation. London: University College.

_____ . 2002b. Diatonic music in Greece: a reassessment of its antiquity. Mnemosyne 56.1: 669-702.

Gadalla, Moustafa. 2002. Egyptian Rhythm: The Heavenly Melodies. Greensboro NC: Tehuti Research Foundation.

Gann K., "An Introduction to Historical Tunings", and "Just Intonation Explained", both available at http://home.earthlink.net/~kgann.html.

Godwin, Jocelyn. 1987. Harmonies of Heaven and Earth: The Spiritual Dimensions of Music from Antiquity to the Avant-Garde. London: Thames and Hudson.

_____. 1993. The Harmony of the Spheres; A Sourcebook of the Pythagorean Tradition in Music. Rochester,VT: Inner Traditions International.

Guthrie, Kenneth S., ed. 1987. The Pythagorean Sourcebook and Library; An Anthology of Ancient Writings Which Relate to Pythagoras and Pythagorean Philosophy. Grand Rapids MI: Phanes Press.

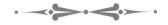

Haase, Rudolf. 1969. Geschichte des harmonikalen Pythagoreismus. Wien: Lafite.

_____. 1974. Aufsätze zur harmonikalen Naturphilosophie. Graz: Akademische Druck.

Hall, RW and Josic, K. "The Mathematics of Musical Instruments", http://www.sju.edu/~rhall/newton/, 2000.

Haramein N and Rauscher EA. The origin of spin: A consideration of torque and coriolis forces in Einstein's field equations and Grand Unification Theory. Special Issue of the *Noetic Journal* Vol. 6 No. 1-4, June, 2005, pp. 143-162. ISSN 1528-3739.

Haynes, Raymond, et al. 1996. Explorers of the Southern Sky: A History of Australian Astronomy. Cambridge: Cambridge University Press.

Helmholtz, H. On the Sensations of Tone, New York: Dover Publications, Inc., 1954; originally published 1885.

Hendricks, John D. Prosperity God's Way. Oviedo, Florida: Christian Research and Fellowship, 1997.

Hollander, John, 1970. The Untuning of the Sky: Ideas of music in English poetry, 1500-1700. New York: Norton.

http://www.fredonia.edu/department/math/MasterSyl/MATH/math307_master.html

Huffman, Carl A. 1993. Philolaus of Croton: Pythagorean and Presocratic. Cambridge: Cambridge University Press.

Isherwood, Robert M. 1973. Music in the Service of the King: France in the Seventeenth Century. Ithaca: Cornell University Press.

Kayser, Hans. 1978. Akroasis: The Theory of World Harmonics. Trans. Robert Lilienfeld. Boston: Plowshare Press.

_____. 1968. Die Harmonie der Welt. Wien: Lafite.

_____.1958. Paestum: Die Nomoi der drei altgriechischen Tempel zu Paestum. Heidelberg: Lambert Schneider.

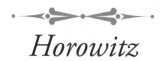
Kilmer, Anne D., et al. 1976. Sounds from Silence: Recent discoveries in ancient Near Eastern music. Berkeley: Bit Enki.

Lawlor, Robert. 1991. Voices of the First Day: Awakening in the Aboriginal Dreamtime. Rochester, VT: Inner Traditions International.

Levarie, Siegmund. 1976. Introduction to The Myth of Invariance: The Origin of the Gods, Mathematics and Music from the Rg Veda to Plato. New York: Nicolas Hays.

Lovelock, James E. 1979. Gaia: A new look at life on Earth. Oxford: Oxford University Press.

May, M. "Did Mozart Use the Golden Section?" American Scientist, March-April 1996; available at http://www.sigmaxi.org/amsci/Issues/Sciobs96/Sciobs96-03MM.html.

McClain, Ernest G. 1976. The Myth of Invariance: The Origin of the Gods, Mathematics and Music from the Rg Veda to Plato. New York: Nicolas Hays.

_____. 1978. The Pythagorean Plato: Prelude to the Song Itself. Stony Brook NY: Nicolas Hays.

_____. 1979. "Chinese Cyclic Tunings in Late Antiquity", *Ethnomusicology*, V. 23, n2.

_____. 1985. The bronze chime bells of the Marquis of Zeng: Babylonian biophysics in Ancient China. Journal of Social and Biological Structures 8: 147-173.

Michaelides, Solon. 1978. The Music of Ancient Greece: An encyclopaedia. London: Faber and Faber.

Michell, John. 1988. The Dimensions of Paradise: the proportions and symbolic numbers of ancient cosmology. London: Thames and Hudson.

Miller, James L. 1986. Measures of Wisdom: The Cosmic Dance in Classical and Christian Antiquity. Toronto: University of Toronto Press.

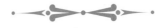
Müller, Hartmut. *Theory of Global Scaling*. Sante Fe, NM: Institute for Space-Energy Research, Leonard Euler, Ltd, and Global Scaling Applications, Inc., 2002.

Mumford, Lewis. 1967. The Myth of the Machine: Technics and Human Development. London: Secker & Warburg.

Neuwirth, E. "Designing a Pleasing Sound Mathematically", Mathematics Magazine, Vol. 74, No. 2, April 2001.

Pont, Graham. 1997. Transforming Total Art. Transforming Art 4, 3: 47-56.

Pont, Graham. "Philosophy and Science of Music in Ancient Greece: Predecessors of Pythagoras and their Contribution", Nexus Network Journal, vol. 6 no. 1 (Spring 2004), See: http://www.nexusjournal. com/filename.html and http://www.emis.de/journals/NNJ/Pont-v6n1.html

Preziosi, Donald. 1983. Minoan Architectural Design: Formation and Signification. Berlin: Mouton.

Ptolemy, Harmonics, translated and commentary by Jon Solomon, Koninklijke Brill NV, Leiden, The Netherlands, 2002.

Purce, Jill. 1974. The Mystic Spiral: Journey of the Soul. London: Thames and Hudson.

Rodin, Marko. The Rodin Project. Available online at: http://rodin-project.com

Roederer, JG. The Physics and Psychophysics of Music, New York: Springer Verlag, 1995.

Rudhyar, Dane. 1982. The Magic of Tone and the Art of Music. Boulder Co: Shambhala Publications.

Sachs, Curt. 1937. World History of the Dance. New York: Norton.

Scholtz, KP. "Algorithmis for Mapping Diatonic Keyboard Tunings and Temperaments", Music Theory Online, http://www.smt.ucsb. edu/mto/issues/mto.98.4.4/mto98.4.4.scholtz.html.

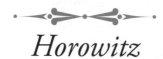

Schulter M. Pythagorean Tuning, http://www.medieval.org/emfaq/harmony/pyth5.html.

Schwaller de Lubicz, R.A. 1977. The Temple in Man: Sacred Architecture and the Perfect Man. Trans. R. and D. Lawlor. New York: Inner Traditions International.

Seidenberg, Abraham. 1962. The ritual origin of geometry. Archive for History of Exact Sciences 1, 488-527.

_____. 1981. The ritual origin of the circle and square. Archive for History of Exact Sciences 25: 269-327.

Sheldrake, Rupert. 1988. The Presence of the Past: Morphic resonance and the habits of nature. London: Fontana.

Shepard, M. Simple Flutes: How to Play or Make a Flute of Bamboo, Wood, Clay, Metal, Plastic, or Anything Else, Simple Productions, Los Angeles, 2001; available as an e-book at www.markshep.com/flute.

Spitzer, Leo. 1963. Classical and Christian Ideas of World Harmony: Prolegomena to an Interpretation of the Word "Stimmung". Baltimore: Johns Hopkins Press.

Stewart, I. Another Fine Math You've Got Me Into, New York: W. H. Freeman and Co., 1992.

Szabó, Árpád. 1978. The beginnings of Greek mathematics. Dordrecht: D. Reidel.

Teilhard de Chardin, Pierre. 1955. The Phenomenon of Man. Trans. Bernard Wall. London: Collins.

Van der Waerden, B.L. 1983. Geometry and Algebra in Ancient Civilizations. Berlin: Springer-Verlag.

Vatsyayan, Kapila. 1983. The Square and the Circle of the Indian Arts. New Delhi: Rolli Books.

Vitruvius. 1999. Ten Books on Architecture. Ingrid Rowland and Thomas Howe, eds. Cambridge: Cambridge University Press.

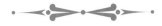

Xenakis I. Formalized Music: Thought and Mathematics in Music, Pendragon Press, Hillsdale, NY, 1992.

Zarlino G. The Art of Counterpoint (Part 3 of Le Institutioni Harmoniche), 1558, translated by Guy A. Marco and Claude V. Palisca, New York: Da Capo Press, 1983.

Zatorre, RJ and Krumhansl, CI. "Mental Models and Musical Minds", Science, 13 December 2002, Vol. 298.

Recommended Textbooks:

1. Math and Music: Harmonious Connections, by Trudi Hammel Garland and Charity Vaughan Kahn, Dale Seymour Publications, 1995.

2. Emblems of Mind: The Inner Life of Music and Mathematics, by Edward Rothstein, Avon Books, 1995.

3. Temperament: The Idea that Solved Music's Greatest Riddle, by Stuart Isacoff, Alfred A. Knopf, 2001.

4. MATH 307 Reader, a compilation of articles, excerpts, and handouts, available at the Connections Bookstore.

5. H.F. Cohen, Quantifying Music: The Science of Music at the First Stage of the Scientific Revolution, 1580-1650, D. Reidel Publishing Co., 1984.

6. Erich Neuwirth, Musical Temperaments, text and CD, Springer-Verlag/Wien, New York, 1997.

7. Philip Wheelwright, The Presocratics, Odyssey Press, ITT Bobbs-Merrill Educational Publishing Company, Inc., Indianapolis, 1985.

8. A.E. Taylor, Aristotle on his Predecessors, The Open Court Publishing Company, London, 1949.

9. Nan Cooke Carpenter, Music in the Medieval and Renaissance Universities, University of Oklahoma Press, Norman, 1958.

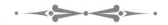

10. Raymond J. Seeger, Galileo Galilei, His Life and His Works, Pergamon Press, Oxford, 1966.

11. John Backus, The Acoustical Foundations of Music, 2nd ed., WW Norton and Company, Inc., New York, 1977.

12. Thomas D. Rossing, The Science of Sound, 2nd ed., Addison-Wesley Publishing Company, 1990; accompanying CD.

13. Calvin M. Bower (translator), Boethius' The Principles of Music, an Introduction, Translation, and Commentary, Ph.D. dissertation, School of Music, George Peabody College for Teachers, 1966.

14. Edward A. Lippman, Musical Thought in Ancient Greece, Columbia University Press, New York, 1964.

15. Richard Hope (translator), Aristotle's Metaphysics, Columbia University Press, New York, 1952.

16. Oliver Strunk, Source Readings in Music History, from Classical Antiquity through the Romantic Era, W.W. Norton and Company, Inc., New York, 1950.

17. J. A. Philip, Pythagoras and Early Pythagoreanism, University of Toronto Press, 1966.

18. Philip Merlan, From Platonism to Neoplatonism, 2nd ed., Martinus Nijhoff, The Hague, 1960.

19. Sir James Jeans, Science and Music, Dover Publications, Inc., New York, 1968; originally published 1937.

20. Dover Art Library. LEONARDO Drawings: 60 Illustrations. Minela, NY: Dover Publications, Inc. 1980.

[1] An erudite and forthright critic of the Greeks was William Chappell (1809-1888): "There is no longer room to doubt that the entire Greek system was mainly derived from Egypt, Phoenicia, Babylon, or other countries of more ancient civilization than Greece" [Chappell 1874, 1].

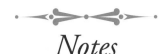

Notes

[2] [Cornford 1952, 107ff]. Europe's last distinguished representative of this ancient tradition was probably St Francis of Assisi, whose fits of ecstasy and sermon to the birds (c.1220) are unmistakably shamanic. So are Socrates' 'daemon' (or 'inner voice') and his trances.

[3] From Abaris, his 'Hyperborean' disciple, Pythagoras obtained a golden arrow that, like the witch's broom, enabled him to fly and appear the same day in two towns separated by 'a journey of many days'. See Guthrie 1987, 90-91, 128.

[4] The story of Pythagoras meditating 'the greater part of day and night' in a cave outside the city of Samos [Guthrie 1987, 62] recalls another familiar practice of the shamans. return to text

[5] Lawlor, C.F. 1991, 48. It should be kept in mind that Chatwin's influential book, though based on personal experience of Aboriginal Australia, is a work of literary rather than strictly scientific anthropology.

[6] Some years ago I applied for a major research grant to conduct a comparative and historical study of the Aboriginal Corroboree as the 'indigenous Australian opera'. The application was referred to the two most eminent female anthropologists in the country, one of whom gave the project a top rating for its originality and national significance; the other (who happened to have been trained by the same philosophers who taught me) utterly damned the whole idea, especially with the revelation that I had never attended a corroboree (except, that is, of the imported kind).

[7] They also report a perfect example of 'As above so below': 'Central Australian tribes believed that the Milky Way divided the sky people into two tribes and hence served as a perpetual reminder that a similar division of lands should be observed by local neighbouring tribes' (loc. cit.).

[8] Op cit., Miller, 1986, especially Foreword and Chapter 1. and Doczi 1994, Chapter 4.

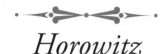

[9] For a concise summary of the Pythagorean doctrine and the ancient literary evidence, see Michaelides, 1978,129-30.

[10] Gadalla 2002, 22-3 claims the harmony of the spheres (that is, the 'planetary scale', the melodious movement of the classical 'planets', from Earth to Saturn, and including the Sun and Moon, in the proportions of a diatonic scale) as a purely Egpytian discovery. Fabre d'Olivet had long ago reached a similar conclusion. See Godwin 1993, 347ff.

[11] I once speculated that the root meaning of 'section cut off' referred to the sectio canonis or division of the monochord but this hypothesis over-simplifies what must have been a very protracted history of human invention and social development. Following Abraham Seidenberg, I now think it more likely that the 'tem-' words originally referred to ritual or liturgical procedures of 'cutting off' or delineating sections of space and time as, for example, in the timing of festivals or the reservation of sacred enclosures. Much later the 'tem-' vocabulary was extended to musical theory, as in the terms 'temper' and 'temperament'.

[12] 'In the seventh century... Sparta was the most important musical center of Greece' (Comotti 1989, 17).

[13] The classical Greek music theorists concentrated their efforts on the measurement of melody and rhythm and the development of a fairly precise notation for both. (See: Comotti 1989, 110-20.) Their greatest achievement (the significance of which has often been overlooked) was probably the quantitative analysis of the various tribal or regional 'modes' and the codification of their distinctive rhythms and accents. While the Greeks relied heavily on their predecessors in speculative music and tuning systems, their empirical and mathematical studies of contemporary song and dance were the beginning of comparative musicology in the West.

[14] John Curtis Franklin has recently thrown new light on the influence of 'Mesopotamian diatony' on Greek music during the 'orientalising period' (c.750-650 BC). (See also: Franklin 2002a, 2002b.)

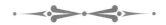

LOVE The Real Da Vinci CODE

[15] Even so, one might wonder how long it will take the recent progress in harmonic studies to affect the structure and content of academic courses in music, architecture, mathematics, aesthetics, cultural history, etc.

16] Regarding the pentacle, the Saint Christopher's cross, and the holy grail quest, Dan Brown's book accurately detailed some of the specifics regarding the "power of symbols." His hero, Harvard Professor of Religious Symbology, and author of the books *The Symbology of Secret Sects, The Art of the Illuminati, The Lost Language of Ideograms,* said "The pentacle is representative of the *female* half of all things—a concept religious historians call the 'sacred feminine' or the 'divine goddess.'. . . . [T]he pentacle symbolizes Venus—the goddess of female sexual Love and beauty. . . .

"Early religion was based on the divine order of Nature. The goddess Venus and the planet Venus were one and the same. The goddess had a place in the night-time sky and was known by many names—Venus, the Eastern Star, Ishtar, Astarte—all of them powerful female concepts with ties to Nature and Mother Earth. . . . [T]he planet Venus traced a perfect pentacle acros the ecliptic sky every eight years. . . . [T]he pentacle's true origins were actually quite godly.

"'I assure you,' Landon said, 'despite what you see in the movies, the pentacle's demonic interpretation is historically accurate. The original feminine meaning is correct, but the symbolism of the pentacle has been distorted over the millennia. In this case, through bloodshed.' (pp. 36-37, *The Da Vinci Code.*)

[17] "[T] ratios of line segments in a pentacle all equal PHI [1.618, the 'Divine Proportion.' PHI is the] fundamental building block in nature. Plants, animals, and even human beings all possess dimensional properties that adhere with . . . the ratio PHI to 1. . . . [T]he number PHI must have been preordained by the Creator of the universe. . . . Da Vinci was the first to show that the human body is literally made of building blocks whose proportional rations always equal PHI. . . . My friends, each of you is a walking tribute to the *Divine Proportion.* . . . God's hand is evident in Nature. . . . [T]he

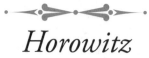
ratios of line segments in a pentacle all equal PHI, making this symbol the *ultimate* expression of Divine Proportion. For this reason, the five-pointed star has always been the symbol for beauty and perfection associated with the goddess and the sacred feminine."(p. 96)

[18] *Anagrams*, such as those found by Michael MacKay adorning American coins and currency, are historically linked to mystical teachings of the Kabbala. Rearranged letters in Hebrew words were used to message new meanings. According to The Da Vinci Code, "French kings throughout the Renaissance were so convinced that anagrams held magic power that they appointed royal anagrammatists to help them make better decisions by analyzing words in important documents. The Romans actually referred to the study of anagrams as *ars magna*—'the great art.'"

[19] Michael K. Mackay, the cryptologist that did an excellent job decoding masses amounts of information hidden in America's currency and coins, is available for contact as follows: P. O. Box 1171, Foresthill, CA 95631; E-mail: iddod2002@yahoo.com; telephone: 530-367-4362.

[20] Psycho-acoustic entrainment expert Joshua Leeds's website is: http://www.incrediblehorizons.com/psychoacoustics.html)

[21] Moses's Hebrew name literally means "Saving from the water." He was spared from Pharaoh's dictate to kill Hebrew first born males by being hidden in the Nile river. This is symbolic of "saving" humanity through the water.

[22] Information on the Medici family derives from seveal sources including http://www.pbs.org/empires/medici/medici/index.html.

ANSWER KEY:

Chapter 6: Exercise #3—9 is "completion"; #4—a. "Sion" as in Priory of Sion; b. 144,000 sing new song for "completion;" c. the forehead is the site of the pineal gland, the electromagnetic processing station of the forebrain regulating all neurology and endocrinology; d. water(s), (Note: *thunder* comes from lightening or electrical current flows between earth and "heaven," and *harps* are stringed instruments that relay sound waves of vibrational energy.)

Chapter 7: Exercise #2—The hidden number code or pattern is: 9-1-3-6-1-6-3-1-9. Notice the 1s exclusively separate the 3s, 6s, and 9s; #3—a. 3-6-9; b. 6-3-9; c. not really, highly unique, all 9s; d. yes; e. yes!

Chapter 9: Exercise #1—8s; #2—a-c) 666; #3: 9; #4: designers of alpha-numeric code; #5) alpha-numeric code; 6) 3, 6, 8 and 9; 7) 144,000.

Chapter 10: Exercise #2—a) god; b) live; c) devil; d) on; e) s[a]y or se[e]; f) DNA; g) mor[ph].

Chapter 11: Exercise #1a) O; b) O; c) ℧ ; d) 9 ; e) 3; f) 6; g) ⤭ #3—a) 345678; 912345; 678912

Chapter 12: Exercise #3—1,2,4,8,7,5 repeats to eternity.

Chapter 14: The sequence is—1 7 4, 2 8 5, 3̲ 9 6̲, 4 1̲ 7̲, 5̲ 2 8̲, 6 3̲ 9 , 7 4̲ 1, 8 5̲ 2̲ , 9 6 3.